D1442779

The Black Death

The Black Death

Other books in the History Firsthand series:

The Black Death

Thomas Streissguth, *Book Editor*

Daniel Leone, *President*
Bonnie Szumski, *Publisher*
Scott Barbour, *Managing Editor*
David M. Haugen, *Series Editor*

GREENHAVEN
PRESS®

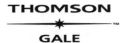

THOMSON

GALE

San Diego • Detroit • New York • San Francisco • Cleveland
New Haven, Conn. • Waterville, Maine • London • Munich

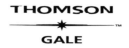

LIBRARY OF CONGRESS CATALOGING-IN-PUBLICATION DATA

The black death / Thomas Streissguth, book editor.
    p. cm. — (History firsthand)
  Includes bibliographical references and index.
  ISBN 0-7377-2253-3 (pbk. : alk. paper) — ISBN 0-7377-2252-5 (lib. : alk. paper)
    1. Plague—History. I. Streissguth, Thomas, 1958– . II. Series.
RC172.B56 2004
362.19'69232'094—dc21

                                       2003055109

Contents

Chapter 1: The Plague in the Ancient World

Chapter 2: The Spread of the Black Death

shelter from the plague, however, had little effect, nor did the blessings of the pope himself prevent the deaths of millions. The arrival of plague in the papal city of Avignon is described firsthand in this poignant and anonymous letter.

Chapter 3: Explaining and Contending with the Plague

for mercy, a sect of penitents known as the flagellants began traveling through Europe, publicly scourging themselves for the sake of preventing God's wrath.

Chapter 5: The Plague Year in London

  The English writer Daniel Defoe, well known in
  modern times for his novel *Robinson Crusoe*, described a devastating outbreak of plague that took
  place in London in 1665. In this extract from his fictional book *A Journal of the Plague Year*, Defoe
  draws on eyewitness accounts to sketch frightening
  and poignant scenes in a London neighborhood.

  A noted English diarist, Samuel Pepys wrote of his
  everyday experiences, detailing his meals, his conver-
  sations, his business dealings, his family life, and his
  sleeping habits. In 1665, with the rest of London's inhabitants, Pepys experienced a frightening visitation
  of the plague.

Foreword

In his preface to a book on the events leading to the Civil War, Stephen B. Oates, the historian and biographer of Abraham Lincoln, John Brown, and other noteworthy American historical figures, explained the difficulty of writing history in the traditional third-person voice of the biographer and historian. "The trouble, I realized, was the detached third-person voice," wrote Oates. "It seemed to wring all the life out of my characters and the antebellum era." Indeed, how can a historian, even one as prominent as Oates, compete with the eloquent voices of Daniel Webster, Abraham Lincoln, Harriet Beecher Stowe, Frederick Douglass, and Robert E. Lee?

Oates's comment notwithstanding, every student of history, professional and amateur alike, can name a score of excellent accounts written in the traditional third-person voice of the historian that bring to life an event or an era and the people who lived through it. In *Battle Cry of Freedom*, James M. McPherson vividly re-creates the American Civil War. Barbara Tuchman's *The Guns of August* captures in sharp detail the tensions in Europe that led to the outbreak of World War I. Taylor Branch's *Parting the Waters* provides a detailed and dramatic account of the American Civil Rights Movement. The study of history would be impossible without such guiding texts.

Nonetheless, Oates's comment makes a compelling point. Often the most convincing tellers of history are those who lived through the event, the eyewitnesses who recorded their firsthand experiences in autobiographies, speeches, memoirs, journals, and letters. The Greenhaven Press History Firsthand series presents history through the words of first-person narrators. Each text in this series captures a significant historical era or event—the American Civil War, the

Great Depression, the Holocaust, the Roaring Twenties, the 1960s, the Vietnam War. Readers will investigate these historical eras and events by examining primary-source documents, authored by chroniclers both famous and little known. The texts in the History Firsthand series comprise the celebrated and familiar words of the presidents, generals, and famous men and women of letters who recorded their impressions for posterity, as well as the statements of the ordinary people who struggled to understand the storm of events around them—the foot soldiers who fought the great battles and their loved ones back home, the men and women who waited on the breadlines, the college students who marched in protest.

The texts in this series are particularly suited to students beginning serious historical study. By examining these firsthand documents, novice historians can begin to form their own insights and conclusions about the historical era or event under investigation. To aid the student in that process, the texts in the History Firsthand series include introductions that provide an overview of the era or event, timelines, and bibliographies that point the serious student toward key historical works for further study.

The study of history commences with an examination of words—the testimony of witnesses who lived through an era or event and left for future generations the task of making sense of their accounts. The Greenhaven Press History Firsthand series invites the beginner historian to commence the process of historical investigation by focusing on the words of those individuals who made history by living through it and recording their experiences firsthand.

Introduction: Contending with the Black Death

In the fall of 1347 a small fleet of Genoese trading ships arrived at the docks of Messina, Sicily. The ships had traveled from Kaffa, a port on the northern reaches of the Black Sea. Since leaving Kaffa, their crews had been struggling against a terrifying, deadly disease. At first, the victims suffered fever, chills, headaches, and nausea. Painful tumors appeared around the lymph nodes in their armpits and groins. Hunger, lethargy, and attacks of mania and panic lasted for several days, followed by death.

The Black Death had arrived in Europe. Before the epidemic of bubonic and pneumonic plague died out three years later, it would kill more than one-third of the continent's population. Entire villages would disappear. Monasteries and manors would be transformed into ghost towns. Serfs would abandon the lands their families had worked for generations, and cultivated fields would return to wilderness. Those who survived would live in a changed society. The plague would alter their view of religion and science, their social customs, their economic life, and their practice of the healing arts.

The Terror of the Plague

The people of fourteenth-century Europe had no notion of the cause of plagues. They could only wait helplessly as terrible omens appeared and the mysterious illness spread. At first, rats and domestic animals would die by the hundreds in the streets and houses. Soon afterward, the first reports of a human victim would spread. Many churches raised black flags to warn of the impending disaster, and panic set in as more people fell ill. According to the chronicler of the Neuberg monastery in Austria,

> The inhabitants, frantic with terror, ordered that no foreigners should stay in the inns, and that the merchants by whom the pestilence was being spread should be compelled to leave the area immediately. The deadly plague reigned everywhere, and once populous cities, because of the death of their inhabitants, now kept their houses firmly shut so that no one could break in and steal the possessions of the dead.[1]

Townspeople who could, fled to the countryside, believing that isolation would spare them. Those who could not flee shut themselves up in their houses. They could do nothing but wait. The plague would run its course in a few months, moving from town to town, then disappear from the region as mysteriously as it had appeared.

Origins of the Plague

Modern scientists believe that the Black Death of the fourteenth century began in central Asia and Mongolia (where the plague bacillus remains endemic among rats, marmots, squirrels, and other small mammals). In the 1330s a warming of the climate in this region drove the animal plague hosts into closer proximity to humans. From human settlements and nomad camps, the plague spread along the trade routes linking central Asia with Black Sea ports that had been established by wealthy European cities such as Genoa and Venice. Ships traveling back to Europe from these ports helped transmit the disease westward.

The spread of the Black Death, however, was also in part a deliberate act of warfare—a medieval version of bioterrorism. The Tatars, a nomadic people of central Asia and the plains of Russia, staged frequent raids on trading caravans and on the Black Sea towns. At one point, during a siege of the port of Kaffa, the Tatars launched diseased animals over the walls of the city in order to kill or drive away the defenders. These animal carcasses carried the plague bacillus. Genoese ships that fled Kaffa during the siege sailed for home, unaware that they were bringing a deadly cargo of plague back to Sicily in the fall of 1347.

Men of Learning Offer Explanations

Once the plague landed in Europe, the devastation was immediate. Civic leaders in southern Europe had no idea that this destroyer of towns had been imported; worse than that, they had no idea how to stop the disease. Mayors and monarchs turned to men of science, men of medicine, and church leaders to provide an explanation. These learned men had never seen anything like the Black Death before. They could only speculate as to its cause, and their speculations seemed to many quite useless. The only explanation that satisfied both learned and ignorant men was that the disease was a divine punishment. For the sins of the world, God was striking down humanity without mercy. The seeming randomness of its victims was a manifestation of God's unknowable will.

In the Middle Ages, the University of Paris was considered to be the capital of learning in western Europe, the place where the most knowledgeable men of the continent gathered. The kings of France often turned to these men for information and advice. As the disease began to ravage his kingdom, and then overcome the capital of Paris, the present king, Philip VI, again sought out the Paris faculty. In October 1348 they offered their explanation for the plague. After serious study, the university elite asserted that an evil conjunction of the stars and planets had corrupted the air. In their report, the faculty wrote out their conclusion:

Although major pestilential illnesses can be caused by the corruption of water or food, as happens at times of famine and infertility, yet we still regard illnesses proceeding from the corruption of air as much more dangerous. This is because bad air is more noxious than food or drink in that it can penetrate quickly to the heart and lungs to do its damage. We believe that the present epidemic or plague has arisen from air corrupt in its substance, and not changed in its attributes. . . . What happened was that the many vapours which had been corrupted at the time of the conjunction were drawn up from the earth and water, and were then mixed with the air and spread abroad by frequent gusts of wind in the wild southerly gales, and because of these alien vapours, which they carried on the winds corrupted the air in its substance, and are still doing so.[2]

Like university lecturers, professional astrologers were held in high regard as men of learning in medieval Europe. They also explained the plague as the result of an unlucky alignment of the planets and stars in the twelve signs of the zodiac. Because the earth and the heavens above were part of one unity, the reasoning went, the movements of planets must have their effects in the terrestrial world. The complex calculations of astrologers, and their many arcane terms and explanations, seemed to make them experts in a very sophisticated field of knowledge. Their most ardent believers were Europe's leading citizens—nobles, royalty, and church leaders—many of whom kept private astrologers in their households.

The scientists and philosophers of the day made a great variety of other educated guesses. To some, earthquakes had released miasmic vapors into the air, which then carried the disease on the currents of the wind. To the man known as the Montpelier physician, the Black Plague was transmitted by bad spirits that pass from one glance to another, a very deadly occurrence of the "evil eye":

> The greater strength of this epidemic and, as it were, instantaneous death is when the aerial spirit going out of the eyes of the sick strikes the eyes of the well person standing near and looking at the sick, especially when they are in agony; for then the poisonous nature of that member passes from one to the other, killing the other.[3]

Whatever the scientific explanation might be, these men offered very little in the way of remedies. Victims were simply isolated. If they were lucky, they kept company with courageous family members who stayed behind to care for them. Millions of others died alone, however, when their entire households—parents, spouses, children—fled in terror. Many healthy people, finding themselves inside a house with a plague victim, found themselves walled into their homes by the authorities. They were left to starve to death or, as was more likely, die of the plague.

The Plague Moves North

In 1347 the plague followed the Rhone River valley and other important water routes to circulate through France. From there, it spread to northern Germany, the Low Countries (modern Belgium and Holland), then to Scandinavia. As the epidemic reached England in the summer of 1348, it picked up strength. Bristol, Plymouth, Southampton, London, and other port towns were struck first. The disease moved inland, skipping from one village to the next and making its way north to Scotland. Livestock died by the thousands in the fields, their rotting and revolting carcasses untouched by birds of prey. Fields and pastures went untended and unharvested. A shortage of workers made the economy falter, but those left alive could demand higher wages. Thus, the economy of England, and the rest of Europe, was permanently disrupted and transformed by the Black Death.

Physicians Face the Plague

As the intellectual elite could offer no remedy for the rapidly spreading disease, doctors, who held a lower standing than astrologers or university lecturers, were left to confront the plague and its ugly symptoms. They went about the cities, visiting one plague-stricken house after another. Many physicians wore distinctive costumes and masks that marked their unpleasant vocation, and their repeated visits to a neighborhood signaled that the plague had come.

Most physicians saw their first duty in securing the patient's confession to a member of the clergy, as the purge of sins and the healing of the soul were held all-important. For the treatment of plague symptoms, doctors prescribed a variety of medicines, certain very unpleasant foods and diets, the use of aromatic spices, bleeding, fervent prayer and religious devotion, as well as the total isolation of their patients. They lit fires both within and in front of the houses of their patients to counteract the effects of evil vapors. For their healthy clients, doctors advised immediate flight. All those who could afford to follow this prescription did so.

When it was clear that their own remedies had no effect, Europe's physicians also took themselves out of harm's way. Many abandoned cities and towns, and several of those who remained behind refused to see plague patients at all.

There were committed physicians as well, who not only treated the sick but who also willingly handled the infected bodies of the dead to investigate the nature of the disease. According to an account of an anonymous writer, who witnessed the Black Death in the city of Avignon, France,

> Examinations have been made by doctors in many cities of Italy, and also in Avignon, by order of the Pope, in order to discover the origin of this disease. Many dead bodies have been thus opened and dissected, and it is found that all who have died thus suddenly have had their lungs infected and have spat blood. . . . There is another form of the sickness, however, at present running its course concurrently with the first; that is, certain aposthumes [tumors] appear under both arms, and by these also people quickly die.[4]

The doctors defying custom and religious sanctions by dissecting bodies were discovering that the victims of the Black Death were dying of two different plague forms,

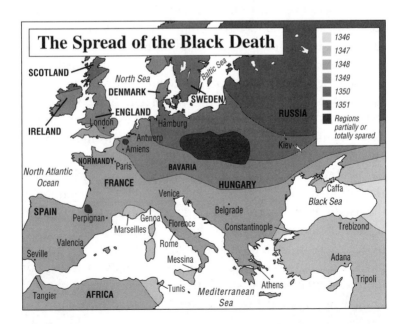

The Spread of the Black Death

1346
1347
1348
1349
1350
1351
Regions partially or totally spared

SCOTLAND
North Sea
Baltic Sea
DENMARK
SWEDEN
ENGLAND
London
Hamburg
RUSSIA
IRELAND
Antwerp
Amiens
Kiev
NORMANDY
Paris
BAVARIA
North Atlantic Ocean
FRANCE
HUNGARY
Venice
Caffa
Black Sea
SPAIN
Belgrade
Perpignan
Genoa
Florence
Constantinople
Trebizond
Marseilles
Valencia
Rome
Seville
Messina
Adana
Tripoli
Tangier
AFRICA
Tunis
Athens
Mediterranean Sea

known today as the "bubonic" and "pneumonic" variants. Whereas the bubonic form of plague attacked the lymph nodes and was spread only by flea bites, pneumonic plague affected the lungs and could be spread by sneezing and coughing. The pneumonic plague was more contagious; it was always fatal, and it killed more swiftly. A small percentage of bubonic plague victims survived, their immune systems now preventing another infection.

The idea of contagious disease did occur to many physicians in Europe as well as in the Islamic world, where the plague had struck concurrently with the Black Death of Europe. The Arab doctor Ibn Khatimah drew the following astute conclusion:

> That the evil spreads is evident from observation and experience, it having not yet happened that a well man remained long with a sick one without being attacked by the disease. . . . Almost as harmful as the air breathed out by the sick, if not entirely so, are the fumes from their bodies, pieces of clothing, beds and linen on which the sick lay, if they are used again.[5]

The idea of disease spreading from one victim to another was commonly believed, but not completely understood, by medieval doctors. They could not grasp the means of transmission; they believed the malady was received from the glance of another person, the inhalation of malevolent vapors, or poor diet and riotous living that left the body prone to sickness. Most cases of plague were in fact caused by the bite of a nearly invisible flea that used the common domestic black rat as a host. Rats were so ubiquitous in medieval Europe that people of the time paid them little attention. No one guessed that the rat problem could be tied to the spread of disease.

Conditions in Europe Facilitate the Spread of the Plague

There were many other realities of fourteenth-century Europe that made the plague epidemic worse than it might have been. The continent was overcrowded, its cities jammed with people living in unsanitary conditions. The thatch used for roofing and walls, and the straw used for bedding, provided perfect nesting places for rats and their fleas. In addition, general conditions of health and nutrition were poor. For centuries, marshes and forest tracts had been cleared for food production, and yet the food supply could not keep pace with the population growth. The result was a series of devastating famines in the early fourteenth century that left Europeans weak and vulnerable to a disease epidemic.

The people of Europe saw hungry packs of wolves descend on their streets and great clouds of ravens and vultures wheeling in the skies above. In the vivid description of twentieth-century author Andrew Nikiforuk,

> Travelling across Europe during the Great Mortality was an alarming experience. Abandoned ships bobbed across the Mediterranean, drifting from one port to another. . . . In the cities, beggars and other folk gathered around bonfires of orange leaves, camphor and sage that cleansed the air, if nothing else. The plague-weary also watched the latest dance craze, a sort of medieval rap in which peasants dressed up as skeletons. The dancing cadavers coarsely reminded spectators that they would soon be "dead, naked, rotting and stinking" and that "power, honour and riches" meant nothing.[6]

Seeing the disease threaten the end of the world, Europeans went to extremes. Many retreated to total isolation, and some formed small communities that walled themselves off completely from the outside world.

New Sanitary Measures Inspired by the Plague

Those who remained behind in the crowded cities could do little to defend themselves against a sickness they did not understand. A few of the wealthiest and most advanced cities did take some measures to improve sanitation such as burying corpses outside the city walls and placing quarantines on infected homes and buildings.

Many cities established committees of public health to

care for the sick, to oversee the disposal of bodies, and supervise basic sewage and garbage-collection services. Special homes were set aside for plague victims, and quarantine of affected households became more common. Other cities ordered the isolation of patients, the examination of cargoes and ships arriving at city gates and docks, and the guarding of shut-up houses. They banned public fairs and celebrations where large crowds gathered and ordered fumigators to disinfect sick houses with burning pitch and sulphur.

In some places, forward-thinking city officials passed new ordinances in an effort to combat the epidemic. In May 1348 the city of Pistoia, Italy, forbade the entrance into the city of any person or object believed to be a carrier of the plague. The author Marchione di Coppo Stefani described other laws written to deal with the many social disruptions:

> When the mortality stopped, women and men in Florence were unmindful of [traditional modesty concerning] their dress. And ordinances were passed concerning this giving authority to the Judge of the Grascia to enforce these ordinances [dress codes]. . . . It was necessary to put a brake on weddings as well because when they gathered for the betrothal each party brought too many people in order to increase the pomp.[7]

The Plague's Long-Term Effects

In the two short years of major outbreak, the Black Death brought many social and economic innovations to medieval Europe. A shortage of laborers drove up wages and drained the feudal estates of their workers, millions of whom sought a better living in the cities once the plague had passed. By loosening the ties that had bound peasants to the land, the Black Death weakened the semi-independent feudal lords who vied with the kings for power and influence. In this way, the plague brought about a centralization of power in the hands of the monarchs.

The plague also had far-ranging effects on European agriculture and environment. With the population of cultivators in sharp decline, crop fields were replaced by new pastures for herds of sheep and cows. The forests of Europe slowly recovered from centuries of overcutting as well.

The art and science of medicine also underwent changes. At one time, the dissection of bodies was strictly forbidden by the church. After the Black Death, however, these strictures loosened. Doctors made a closer study of the human body, which led to a basic understanding of anatomy, the structure of bone and tissue, and the functions of organs. The art of surgery, once frowned upon, gained respect. The universities of Europe began to establish faculties of medicine devoted to the causes, prevention, and treatment of disease. Doctors, who had never enjoyed much respect in medieval Europe, saw their status begin to rise.

But no social or scientific innovation could overcome the dread of the plague, a fear that would haunt Europe for centuries. The terror of the plague was worsened by the fact that it was invisible, and that its origins and cause were unknown.

Storms, floods, fire, famine, and human enemies could all be fought or avoided. There was no weapon available to combat the unseen plague, and so the people of the Middle Ages looked to their faith for answers, believing themselves guilty of corruption and a spiritual failure that brought on the wrath of God. Andrew Nikiforuk comments that "to the shell-shocked survivors of the plague's visitations, it appeared as though God and His able assistant Nature had conspired to destroy human beings. Just as the modern world can imagine no greater horror than nuclear war, so the medieval world had no measuring stick long enough for the plague."[8]

The Plague Revealed

It would be over five hundred years before the true cause of the bubonic plague would be found. In a pair of laboratories set up in a Hong Kong hospital in 1898, the Japanese scientist Shibasaburo Kitasato and Alexander Yersin, a Swiss physician, would discover that the plague was transmitted by a microscopic bacillus, which is now known as *Yersinia pestis*, carried by fleas. In the twentieth century, bubonic plague was fought by injections of tetracycline and other antibiotics, and in nine out of ten cases the victim survived. Nevertheless, the plague has not been completely eradicated and still is endemic to the wilds of central Asia as well as the western United States.

But for the people of an earlier time, the plague would remain a misunderstood and greatly feared illness. The Black Death that began in the fall of 1347 in Messina would, on many occasions, return to Europe, with the last serious outbreaks occurring in the early eighteenth century. The plague would continue to deal widespread death to the continent's largest and wealthiest cities, confounding doctors and men of science and putting the fear of God into people of all social classes and occupations.

Notes

1. Quoted in Rosemary Horrox, ed., *The Black Death.* Manchester, UK: Manchester University Press, 1994, p. 59.
2. Quoted in Horrox, *The Black Death*, pp. 160–61.
3. Quoted in Anna Montgomery Campbell, *The Black Death and Men of Learning.* New York: Columbia University Press, 1931, p. 61.
4. Quoted in Francis Aidan Gasquet, *The Black Death of 1348 and 1349.* London: George Bell and Sons, 1908, pp. 44–45.
5. Quoted in Geoffrey Marks, "Medieval Medicine's Response to the Black Death," in *The Black Death*, ed. Don Nardo. San Diego: Greenhaven, 1999, p. 62.
6. Andrew Nikiforuk, *The Fourth Horseman: A Short History of Epidemics, Plagues, and Other Scourges.* New York: M. Evans, 1993, p. 46.
7. Marchione di Coppo Stefani, "The Florentine Chronicle," in *The Medieval Sourcebook.* http://jefferson.village.virginia.edu/osheim/marchione.html.
8. Nikiforuk, *The Fourth Horseman*, p. 43.

Chapter 1

The Plague in the Ancient World

Chapter Preface

People have always lived with the scourge of plague. In the ancient world, epidemics were a frequent catastrophe that the natural world had to offer, along with storms, floods, fires, earthquakes, and droughts. In ancient Egypt, in the time of Moses, disease was one of many such "plagues" visited on the land of Egypt. In the common understanding of the time, these plagues could mean only one thing: the wrath of God.

Humans will always seek an explanation for the mysterious workings of the natural world. For the people of the Bible, plagues were explained as a divine punishment. In modern times, those who might dismiss religious belief offer a different explanation for events described in the Bible. According to some theories, the eruption of a volcano on the island of Thira (Santorini) in the Greek Aegean Sea caused a huge cloud of ash to form and move over Egypt, darkening the sky. This ash cloud dropped its contents on the Nile River and the surrounding countryside, bringing pollution and widespread contamination that allowed disease to easily spread.

In classical Athens, a place where reason and philosophy were enshrined in the way of a religion, people again sought to explain a devastating plague that struck the city in 430 B.C. As the writer Thucydides explains in his book on the Peloponnesian War, the plague killed thousands of citizens and soldiers who took shelter within the walls of Athens. The plague was at its worst in the summer, when the weather was hot. For modern science, hot and crowded conditions represent ideal breeding grounds for the spread of contagious disease. For the ancient Athenians, the plague struck as retribution for the city's wealth, laziness, and corruption. The mightiest city in Greece, which had lorded it over the cities of the Aegean region for so long, was justly brought low.

Ten centuries later a plague again occurred in the Greek-speaking world. Known as "Justinian's Plague" for the emperor that then ruled the Byzantine Empire, this epidemic spread from Egypt north to the Levant, Asia Minor, Greece, and the Balkan Peninsula. In the capital city of Constantinople, thousands were dying every day. The best physicians in the realm could do nothing to stop the epidemic or slow it down. As in ancient Athens, Justinian's plague struck just as the empire was reaching the height of its power and influence in the eastern Mediterranean. It would be the worst epidemic in history—until the Black Death of the fourteenth century.

The Plague in Ancient Athens

Thucydides

The Athenian aristocrat Thucydides was elected as a general in 424 B.C., seven years after the beginning of the war between the city of Athens and an alliance of Greek city-states led by Sparta, a town on the Peloponnesus. After suffering a military setback, Thucydides was exiled by the leaders of his city. On his travels he spoke to many civilian and military leaders about the war and began writing a masterful history of the conflict, a work known in modern times as *The Peloponnesian War.*

In the following excerpt, Thucydides describes a devastating disease epidemic that began sweeping through Athens in 430 B.C., the second year of the war. The plague endured for at least three years and considerably weakened the Athenian will to carry on the fight against Sparta. Although Thucydides does not name the disease, from his description of the symptoms some (not all) historians have concluded that the culprit was the same bubonic plague that would return to Europe and the Middle East in the fourteenth century. Others have argued for smallpox, typhus, or the Ebola virus, a hemorrhagic fever endemic to central Africa. Whatever the true name of the Athenian plague, it brought misery, demoralization, and lawlessness to a once-wealthy and proud city that had been the intellectual capital of the ancient Mediterranean.

Thucydides, *The Peloponnesian War.* New York: Random House, 1951.

In the first days of summer the Lacedæmonians [Spartans] and their allies, with two-thirds of their forces as before, invaded Attica [the Athenian homeland], under the command of Archidamus, son of Zeuxidamus, king of Lacedæmon, and sat down and laid waste the country. Not many days after their arrival in Attica the plague first began to show itself among the Athenians. It was said that it had broken out in many places previously in the neigbourhood of Lemnos and elsewhere; but a pestilence of such extent and mortality was nowhere remembered. Neither were the physicians at first of any service, ignorant as they were of the proper way to treat it, but they died themselves the most thickly, as they visited the sick most often; nor did any human art succeed any better. Supplications in the temples, divinations, and so forth were found equally futile, till the overwhelming nature of the disaster at last put a stop to them altogether.

It first began, it is said, in the parts of Ethiopia above Egypt, and thence descended into Egypt and Libya and into most of the king's country. Suddenly falling upon Athens, it first attacked the population in [the Athenian port of] Piræus,—which was the occasion of their saying that the Peloponnesians had poisoned the reservoirs, there being as yet no wells there—and afterwards appeared in the upper city, when the deaths became much more frequent. All speculation as to its origin and its causes, if causes can be found adequate to produce so great a disturbance, I leave to other writers, whether lay or professional; for myself, I shall simply set down its nature, and explain the symptoms by which perhaps it may be recognised by the student, if it should ever break out again. This I can the better do, as I had the disease myself, and watched its operation in the case of others.

How the Plague Attacked

That year then is admitted to have been otherwise unprecedentedly free from sickness; and such few cases as occurred, all determined in this. As a rule, however, there was no ostensible cause; but people in good health were all of a sudden attacked by violent heats in the head, and redness and inflammation in the eyes, the inward parts, such as the throat or tongue, becoming bloody and emitting an unnatural and fetid breath. These symptoms were followed by sneezing and hoarseness, after which the pain soon reached the chest, and produced a hard cough. When it fixed in the stomach, it upset it; and discharges of bile of every kind named by physicians ensued, accompanied by very great distress. In most cases also an ineffectual retching followed, producing violent spasms, which in some cases ceased soon after, in others much later. Externally the body was not very hot to the touch, nor pale in its appearance, but reddish, livid, and breaking out into small pustules and ulcers. But internally it burned so that the patient could not bear to have on him clothing or linen even of the very lightest description; or indeed to be otherwise than stark naked. What they would have liked best would have been to throw themselves into cold water; as indeed was done by some of the neglected sick, who plunged into the rain-tanks in their agonies of unquenchable thirst; though it made no difference whether they drank little or much. Besides this, the miserable feeling of not being able to rest or sleep never ceased to torment them. The body meanwhile did not waste away so long as the distemper was at its height, but held out to a marvel against its ravages; so that when they succumbed, as in most cases, on the seventh or eighth day to the internal inflammation, they had still some strength in them. But if they passed this stage, and the disease descended further into the bowels, inducing a violent ulceration there accompanied by severe diarrhœa, this brought on a weakness which was generally fatal. For the disorder first settled in the head, ran its course from thence through the whole of the body, and even where it did not prove mortal, it still left its mark on the extremities; for it settled in the privy parts, the fingers and the toes, and many escaped with the loss of these, some too with that of their eyes. Others again were seized with an entire loss of memory on their first recovery, and did not know either themselves or their friends.

But while the nature of the distemper was such as to baf-

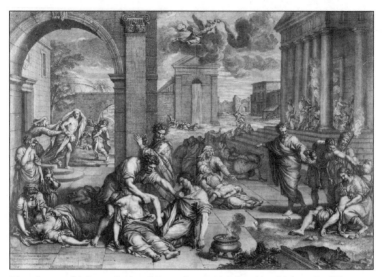

The plague of Athens, depicted here, devastated the city of Athens in 430 B.C., killing one-third of its population.

fle all description, and its attacks almost too grievous for human nature to endure, it was still in the following circumstance that its difference from all ordinary disorders was most clearly shown. All the birds and beasts that prey upon human bodies, either abstained from touching them (though there were many lying unburied), or died after tasting them. In proof of this, it was noticed that birds of this kind actually disappeared; they were not about the bodies, or indeed to be seen at all. But of course the effects which I have mentioned could best be studied in a domestic animal like the dog.

Dejection and Neglect

Such then, if we pass over the varieties of particular cases, which were many and peculiar, were the general features of the distemper. Meanwhile the town enjoyed an immunity from all the ordinary disorders; or if any case occurred, it ended in this. Some died in neglect, others in the midst of every attention. No remedy was found that could be used as a specific; for what did good in one case, did harm in another. Strong and weak constitutions proved equally incapable of resistance, all alike being swept away, although dieted with the utmost precaution. By far the most terrible feature in the malady was the dejection which ensued when any one felt himself sickening, for the despair into which they instantly fell took away their power of resistance, and left them a much easier prey to the disorder; besides which, there was the awful spectacle of men dying like sheep, through having caught the infection in nursing each other. This caused the greatest mortality. On the one hand, if they were afraid to visit each other, they perished from neglect; indeed many houses were emptied of their inmates for want of a nurse: on the other, if they ventured to do so, death was the consequence. This was especially the case with such as made any pretensions to goodness: honour made them unsparing of themselves in their attendance in their friends' houses, where even the members of the family were at last worn out by the moans of the dying, and succumbed to the force of the disaster. Yet it was with those who had recovered from the disease that the sick and the dying found most compassion. These knew what it was from experience, and had now no fear for themselves; for the same man was never attacked twice—never at least fatally. And such persons not only received the congratulations of others, but themselves also, in the elation of the moment, half entertained the vain hope that they were for the future safe from any disease whatsoever.

An aggravation of the existing calamity was the influx from the country into the city, and this was especially felt by the new arrivals. As there were no houses to receive them, they had to be lodged at the hot season of the year in stifling cabins, where the mortality raged without restraint. The bodies of dying men lay one upon another, and half-dead creatures reeled about the streets and gathered round all the fountains in their longing for water. The sacred places also in which they had quartered themselves were full of corpses of persons that had died there, just as they were; for as the disaster passed all bounds, men, not knowing what was to become of them, became utterly careless of everything, whether sacred or profane. All the burial rites before in use were entirely upset, and they buried the bodies as best they could. Many from want of the proper appliances, through so many of their friends having died already, had recourse to the most shameless sepultures [burials]: sometimes getting the start of those who had raised a pile, they threw their own dead body upon the stranger's pyre and ignited it; sometimes they tossed the corpse which they were carrying on the top of another that was burning, and so went off.

Society Breaks Down

Nor was this the only form of lawless extravagance which owed its origin to the plague. Men now coolly ventured on what they had formerly done in a corner, and not just as they pleased, seeing the rapid transitions produced by persons in prosperity suddenly dying and those who before had nothing succeeding to their property. So they resolved to spend quickly and enjoy themselves, regarding their lives and riches as alike things of a day. Perseverance in what men called honour was popular with none, it was so uncertain whether they would be spared to attain the object; but it was settled that present enjoyment, and all that contributed to it, was both honourable and useful. Fear of gods or law of man there was none to restrain them. As for the first, they judged it to be just the same whether they worshipped them or not, as they saw all alike perishing; and for the last, no one expected to live to be brought to trial for his offences, but each felt that a far severer sentence had been already passed upon them all and hung ever over their heads, and before this fell it was only reasonable to enjoy life a little.

Such was the nature of the calamity, and heavily did it weigh on the Athenians; death raging within the city and devastation without. Among other things which they remembered in their distress was, very naturally, the following verse which the old men said had long ago been uttered:

'A Dorian war shall come and with it death.'

So a dispute arose as to whether dearth and not death had not been the word in the verse; but at the present juncture, it was of course decided in favour of the latter; for the people made their recollection fit in with their sufferings. I fancy, however, that if another Dorian war should ever afterwards come upon us, and a dearth should happen to accompany it, the verse will probably be read accordingly. The oracle also which had been given to the Lacedæmonians was now remembered by those who knew of it. When the God was asked whether they should go to war, he answered that if they put their might into it, victory would be theirs, and that he would himself be with them. With this oracle events were supposed to tally. For the plague broke out so soon as the Peloponnesians invaded Attica, and never entering Peloponnese (not at least to an extent worth noticing), committed its worst ravages at Athens, and next to Athens, at the most populous of the other towns. Such was the history of the plague.

Justinian's Plague

Procopius

The Black Death of the fourteenth century did not occur in isolation. There had been many outbreaks of bubonic plague in the ancient world, and there would be more outbreaks in the centuries following the medieval period. One of the worst plague epidemics in history took place in the sixth-century empire ruled by Justinian, the eastern Roman emperor who expanded his domains to include Greece, the Balkan Peninsula, Asia Minor, southern Italy, and the eastern Mediterranean basin.

This plague was documented by the historian Procopius, who described its effects in his work known as the *History of the Wars*. Procopius interrupts his account of Justinian's military conquests with a description of the plague's origins and spread, its terrifying symptoms, and its complete disruption of daily life.

D uring these times there was a pestilence, by which the whole human race came near to being annihilated. Now in the case of all other scourges sent from heaven some explanation of a cause might be given by daring men, such as the many theories propounded by those who are clever in these matters; for they love to conjure up causes which are absolutely incomprehensible to man, and to fabricate outlandish theories of natural philosophy knowing well that they are saying nothing sound but considering it sufficient for them, if they completely deceive by their argument some of those whom they meet and persuade them to their view. But for this calamity it is quite impossible either to express

Procopius, *History of the Wars*, vol. I, translated by H.B. Dewing. Cambridge, MA: Harvard University Press, 1914.

in words or to conceive in thought any explanation, except indeed to refer it to God. For it did not come in a part of the world nor upon certain men, nor did it confine itself to any season of the year, so that from such circumstances it might be possible to find subtle explanations of a cause, but it embraced the entire world, and blighted the lives of all men, though differing from one another in the most marked degree, respecting neither sex nor age.

For much as men differ with regard to places in which they live, or in the law of their daily life, or in natural bent, or in active pursuits, or in whatever else man differs from man, in the case of this disease alone the difference availed naught. And it attacked some in the summer season, others in the winter, and still others at the other times of the year. Now let each one express his own judgment concerning the matter, both sophist [philosopher] and astrologer, but as for me, I shall proceed to tell where this disease originated and the manner in which it destroyed men.

The Disease Spreads from Egypt to Byzantium

It started from the Egyptians who dwell in Pelusium. Then it divided and moved in one direction towards Alexandria and the rest of Egypt, and in the other direction it came to Palestine on the borders of Egypt; and from there it spread over the whole world, always moving forward and travelling at times favorable to it. For it seemed to move by fixed arrangement, and to tarry for a specified time in each country, casting its blight slightingly upon none, but spreading in either direction right out to the ends of the world, as if fearing lest some corner of the earth might escape it. For it left neither island nor cave nor mountain ridge which had human inhabitants; and if it had passed by any land, either not affecting the men there or touching them in indifferent fashion, still at a later time it came back; then those who dwelt round about this land, whom formerly it had afflicted most sorely, it did not touch at all, but it did not remove from the place in question until it had given up its just and proper tale of dead, so as to correspond exactly to the number destroyed at the earlier time among those who dwelt round about. And this disease always took its start from the coast, and from there went up to the interior.

And in the second year it reached Byzantium in the middle of spring, where it happened that I was staying at that time. And it came as follows. Apparitions of supernatural beings in human guise of every description were seen by many persons, and those who encountered them thought that they were struck by the man they had met in this or that part of the body, as it happened, and immediately upon seeing this apparition they were seized also by the disease. Now at first those who met these creatures tried to turn them aside by uttering the holiest of names and exorcising them in other ways as well as each one could, but they accomplished absolutely nothing, for even in the sanctuaries where the most of them fled for refuge they were dying constantly. But later on they were unwilling even to give heed to their friends when they called to them, and they shut themselves up in their rooms and pretended that they did not hear, although their doors were being beaten down, fearing, obviously, that he who was calling was one of those demons.

But in the case of some the pestilence did not come on in this way, but they saw a vision in a dream and seemed to suffer the very same thing at the hands of the creature who stood over them, or else to hear a voice foretelling to them that they were written down in the number of those who were to die. But with the majority it came about that they were seized by the disease without becoming aware of what was coming either through a waking vision or a dream. And they were taken in the following manner. They had a sudden fever, some when just roused from sleep, others while walking about, and others while otherwise engaged, without any regard to what they were doing. And the body showed no change from its previous color, nor was it hot as might be expected when attacked by a fever, nor indeed did any inflammation set in, but the fever was of such a languid sort from its commencement and up till evening that neither to the sick themselves nor to a physician who touched them would it afford any suspicion of danger. It was natural, therefore, that not one of those who had contracted the disease expected to die from it. But on the same day in some cases, in others on the following day, and in the rest not many days later, a bubonic swelling developed; and this took place not only in the particular part of the body which

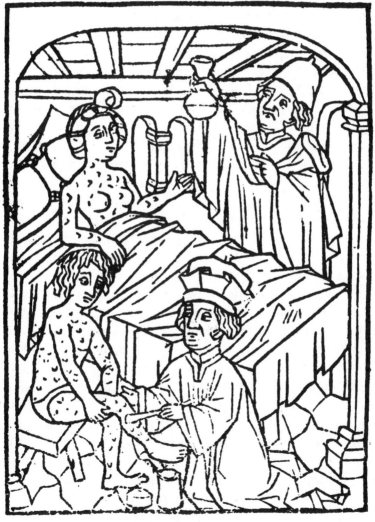

As shown in this woodcut, many ancient physicians treated plague victims with the practice of bloodletting, which was believed to draw out the poisons from the bloodstream.

is called *boubon*, that is, "below the abdomen," but also inside the armpit, and in some cases also beside the ears, and at different points on the thighs.

Comas and Deliriums

Up to this point, then, everything went in about the same way with all who had taken the disease. But from then on very marked differences developed; and I am unable to say whether the cause of this diversity of symptoms was to be found in the difference in bodies, or in the fact that it followed the wish of Him who brought the disease into the world. For there ensued with some a deep coma, with others a violent delirium, and in either case they suffered the characteristic symptoms of the disease. For those who were under the spell of the coma forgot all those who were familiar to them and seemed to lie sleeping constantly. And if anyone cared for them, they would eat without waking, but some also were neglected, and these would die directly through lack of sustenance.

But those who were seized with delirium suffered from insomnia and were victims of a distorted imagination; for they suspected that men were coming upon them to destroy them, and they would become excited and rush off in flight, crying out at the top of their voices. And those who were attending them were in a state of constant exhaustion and had a most difficult time of it throughout. For this reason everybody pitied them no less than the sufferers, not because they were threatened by the pestilence in going near it (for neither physicians nor other persons were found to contract this malady through contact with the sick or with the dead, for many who were constantly engaged either in burying or in attending those in no way connected with them held out in the performance of this service beyond all expectation, while with many others the disease came on without warning and they died straightway); but they pitied them because of the great hardships which they were undergoing. For when the patients fell from their beds and lay rolling upon the floor, they kept putting them back in place, and when they were struggling to rush headlong out of their houses, they would force them back by shoving and pulling against them. And when water chanced to be near, they wished to fall into it, not so much because of a desire for drink (for the most of them rushed into the sea), but the cause was to be found chiefly in the diseased state of their minds. They had also great difficulty in the matter of eating, for they could not easily take food. And many perished through lack of any man to care for them, for they were either overcome by hunger, or threw themselves down from a height. And in those cases where neither coma nor delirium came on, the bubonic swelling became mortified and the sufferer, no longer able to endure the pain, died. And one would suppose that in all cases the same thing would have been true, but since they were not at all in their senses, some were quite unable to feel the pain; for owing to the troubled condition of their minds they lost all sense of feeling.

The Unpredictable Plague

Now some of the physicians who were at a loss because the symptoms were not understood, supposing that the disease centred in the bubonic swellings, decided to investigate the bodies of the dead. And upon opening some of the swellings, they found a strange sort of carbuncle that had grown inside them. Death came in some cases immediately, in others after many days; and with some the body broke out with black pustules about as large as a lentil and these did not survive even one day, but all succumbed immediately. With many also a vomiting of blood ensued without visible cause and straightway brought death. Moreover I am able to declare this, that the most illustrious physicians predicted that many would die, who unexpectedly escaped entirely from suffering shortly afterwards, and that they declared that many would be saved, who were destined to be carried off almost immediately. So it was that in this disease there was no cause which came within the province of human reasoning; for in all cases the issue tended to be something unaccountable. For example, while some were helped by battling, others were harmed in no less degree. And of those who received no care many died, but others, contrary to reason, were saved. And again, methods of treatment showed different results with different patients. Indeed the whole matter may be stated thus, that no device was discovered by man to save himself, so that either by taking precautions he should not suffer, or that when the malady had assailed him he should get the better of it; but suffering came without warning and recovery was due to no external cause. And in the case of women who were pregnant death could be certainly foreseen if they were taken with the disease. For some died through miscarriage, but others perished immediately at the time of birth with the infants they bore. However,

Justinian's Plague Transforms the World

In The Black Death in the Middle East, *author Michael W. Dols describes the far-ranging social and political effects of "Justinian's Plague," the epidemic that flared during the reign of the emperor Justinian in sixth-century Byzantium.*

Wherever the Plague of Justinian may have originated, its description by Procopius is important because it is the first unequivocal account of a bubonic plague epidemic. Procopius observed the distinct symptoms of plague when it ravaged the Byzantine capital of Constantinople. Plague had probably reached the city in the spring of 542, or possibly as early as the autumn of 541, engulfing the lands and peoples of the known world: the Byzantine Empire and the rest of Europe, Persia and the barbarian hinterland. Asia Minor and Egypt particularly were reported to have suffered severely.

The Plague of Justinian may have played a crucial role in the history of the early Middle Ages. Although there is considerable uncertainty about the demographic history of this period, it is fairly certain that the pandemic contributed to the perceptible contraction of Mediterranean population. Professor Russell estimates that the initial plague epidemic of 541–544 reduced the European-Mediterranean population by 20–25 percent and that there was a total decline of about 50–60 percent of the pre-plague population for the period 541–700.

they say that three women in confinement survived though their children perished, and that one woman died at the very time of childbirth but that the child was born and survived.

Now in those cases where the swelling rose to an unusual size and a discharge of pus had set in, it came about that they escaped from the disease and survived, for clearly the acute condition of the carbuncle had found relief in this direction, and this proved to be in general an indication of returning health; but in cases where the swelling preserved its former appearance there ensued those troubles which I have just men-

Despite the slight investigation of the demographic data for the Plague of Justinian, there has been dramatic speculation that the pandemic and its recurrent epidemics were the solvents of classical Mediterranean civilization and were largely responsible for the formation of new political, social, and economic patterns characteristic of the European Middle Ages. According to such speculation, political power gradually shifted to the peoples of northern Europe, who were relatively unaffected by the epidemics, and conversely, plague greatly weakened the Byzantine Empire. Justinian's plan for re-establishing the Roman Empire was wrecked, and the diminished Byzantine armies were unable to defend the extensive frontiers. Hence, there was the successful resurgence of barbarian invasions—the Slavic migrations into the Balkans and Greece, the Lombardic invasion into Italy, and the Berber incursions into Byzantine North Africa. In addition, the pandemic may have had significant economic repercussions comparable to those of the Black Death eight centuries later. The Pirenne Thesis that the advent of Islam produced a rupture in the commerce of the ancient Mediterranean world has been seriously questioned; the discussion of this historical problem should also take into account the consequences of the concomitant drastic decline in Mediterranean population.

Michael W. Dols, *The Black Death in the Middle East.* Princeton, NJ: Princeton University Press, 1977.

tioned. And with some of them it came about that the thigh was withered, in which case, though the swelling was there, it did not develop the least suppuration. With others who survived the tongue did not remain unaffected, and they lived on either lisping or speaking incoherently and with difficulty.

Burying the Dead

Now the disease in Byzantium ran a course of four months, and its greatest virulence lasted about three. And at first the deaths were a little more than the normal, then the mortality rose still higher, and afterwards the tale of dead reached five thousand each day, and again it even came to ten thousand and still more than that. Now in the beginning each man attended to the burial of the dead of his own house, and these they threw even into the tombs of others, either escaping detection or using violence; but afterwards confusion and disorder everywhere became complete. For slaves remained destitute of masters, and men who in former times were very prosperous were deprived of the service of their domestics who were either sick or dead, and many houses became completely destitute of human inhabitants. For this reason it came about that some of the notable men of the city because of the universal destitution remained unburied for many days.

And it fell to the lot of the emperor, as was natural, to make provision for the trouble. He therefore detailed soldiers from the palace and distributed money, commanding Theodorus to take charge of this work; this man held the position of announcer of imperial messages, always announcing to the emperor the petitions of his clients, and declaring to them in turn whatever his wish was. In the Latin tongue the Romans designate this office by the term *Referendarius.* So those who had not as yet fallen into complete destitution in their domestic affairs attended individually to the burial of those connected with them. But Theodorus, by giving out the emperor's money and by making further expenditures from his own purse, kept burying the bodies which were not cared for. And when it came about that all the tombs which had existed previously were filled with the dead, then they dug up all the places about the city one after the other, laid the dead there, each one as he could, and departed; but later on those who were making these trenches, no longer able to keep up with the number of the dying, mounted the towers of the fortifications in Sycae [Asia Minor], and tearing off the roofs threw the bodies there in complete disorder; and they piled them up just as each one happened to fall, and filled practically all the towers with corpses, and then covered them again with their roofs. As a result of this an evil stench pervaded the city and distressed the inhabitants still more, and especially whenever the wind blew fresh from that quarter.

Mending and Unmending One's Ways

At that time all the customary rites of burial were overlooked. For the dead were not carried out escorted by a procession in the customary manner, nor were the usual chants sung over them, but it was sufficient if one carried on his shoulders the body of one of the dead to the parts of the city which bordered on the sea and flung him down; and there the corpses would be thrown upon skiffs in a heap, to be conveyed wherever it might chance. At that time, too, those of the population who had formerly been members of the factions[1] laid aside their mutual enmity and in common they attended to the burial rites of the dead, and they carried with their own hands the bodies of those who were no connections of theirs and buried them. Nay, more, those who in times past used to take delight in devoting themselves to pursuits both shameful and base, shook off the unrighteousness of their daily lives and practiced the duties of religion with diligence, not so much because they had learned wisdom at last nor because they had become all of a sudden lovers of virtue, as it were— for when qualities have become fixed in men by nature or by the training of a long period of time, it is impossible for them to lay them aside thus lightly, except, indeed, some divine influence for good has breathed upon them—but then all, so to

1. Medieval Constantinople was torn by a violent rivalry between groups known as the Blues and Greens.

speak, being thoroughly terrified by the things which were happening, and supposing that they would die immediately, did, as was natural, learn respectability for a season by sheer necessity. Therefore as soon as they were rid of the disease and were saved, and already supposed that they were in security, since the curse had moved on to other peoples, then they turned sharply about and reverted once more to their baseness of hearts and now, more than before, they make a display of the inconsistency of their conduct, altogether surpassing themselves in villainy and in lawlessness of every sort. For one could insist emphatically without falsehood that this disease, whether by chance or by some providence, chose out with exactitude the worst men and let them go free. But these things were displayed to the world in later times.

During that time it seemed no easy thing to see any man in the streets of Byzantium, but all who had the good fortune to be in health were sitting in their houses, either attending the sick or mourning the dead. And if one did succeed in meeting a man going out, he was carrying one of the dead. And work of every description ceased, and all the trades were abandoned by the artisans, and all other work as well, such as each had in hand. Indeed in a city which was simply abounding in all good things starvation almost absolute was running riot. Certainly it seemed a difficult and very notable thing to have a sufficiency of bread or of anything else; so that with some of the sick it appeared that the end of life came about sooner than it should have come by reason of the lack of the necessities of life.

And, to put all in a word, it was not possible to see a single man in Byzantium clad in the *chlamys* [a woolen mantle worn by aristocrats], and especially when the emperor became ill (for he too had a swelling of the groin), but in a city which held dominion over the whole Roman empire every man was wearing clothes befitting private station and remaining quietly at home. Such was the course of the pestilence in the Roman empire at large as well as in Byzantium. And it fell also upon the land of the Persians and visited all the other barbarians besides.

Chapter 2

The Spread of the Black Death

Chapter Preface

In thirteenth-century Europe, the expansion of royal power brought a gradual end to the chaos and conflict that marked the early medieval period. Urban centers such as London, Paris, and Florence flourished through trade. New industries, such as clothmaking, allowed these cities to grow and a middle class of artisans to prosper. But the relatively peaceful and prosperous times also brought overpopulation. The result was a dwindling supply of food, especially in the overcrowded cities. Poor weather hindered the harvests for several years running, and great famines struck in the first two decades of the fourteenth century, when millions of people, many of them young or elderly, died of starvation and disease.

The contagions and hunger weakened the public's health and resistance to disease, making Europeans vulnerable to an epidemic. By the 1340s the bubonic plague was moving west along the caravan routes that linked the ports of the Black Sea to central Asia. When the plague arrived in the Black Sea port of Kaffa, then controlled by the Italian republic of Genoa, the sailors on board a small fleet of ships took sick. In the fall of 1347, when their ships sailed for home, they brought the plague to the port of Messina, Sicily.

The plague spread quickly, from Sicily onto the mainland of Italy, then France and the Low Countries, Germany, and finally the British Isles. The disease moved along common trade and transportation routes, mostly rivers, that merchants depended on to move their goods. The terrifying disease, which attacked with loathsome symptoms and killed within a few days, wiped out families and left entire cities empty, their streets littered with unburied corpses. People took shelter in any way they could, believing that contact with the sick and the dead were the sure means to catch the disease.

In fact, their belief was incorrect. The Black Death was

spread by the bite of fleas that used rats as their hosts and food supply. Rats and fleas were common household pests in the Middle Ages, and nobody paid them much attention. Instead, as in the ancient world, people from all walks of life saw the plague as a form of divine punishment, and only a few cities in Italy actually took preventive sanitation measures. These measures would do little to control rats, and thus did little good. The Black Death would subside by 1349 but return several times to Europe over the next three centuries.

An Emperor Observes the Plague

John VI Cantacuzenos

The Eastern Roman or Byzantine Empire had been the center
of a great plague outbreak in the sixth century. The Byzan-
tines lived astride the busy trading routes between Asia and
Europe, and thus fell easy victim to frequent visitations of the
plague, which had its origins in China and the plains and
deserts of central Asia. According to one ancient historian,
three hundred thousand people died in the capital city of Constantinople during a plague outbreak in 716–717; the Byzantine emperor Constantinos Copronymos died of the same illness in 775.

   After abdicating his throne in 1355, the Byzantine emperor
John VI Cantacuzenos wrote a history of his realm, in which
the following extract describes the plague as it struck the
eastern empire in 1347. The emperor begins by describing the
death of his own son Andronikos from the Black Death.

Upon arrival in Byzantium she [the empress] found Andronikos, the youngest born, dead from the invading
plague, which, starting first from the Hyperborean Scythi-
ans [of the Crimea], attacked almost all the sea coasts of the
world and killed most of their people. For it swept not only
through Pontus [on the Black Sea coast], Thrace and Mace-
donia, but even Greece, Italy and all the islands, Egypt,
Libya, Judaea and Syria, and spread throughout almost the
entire world.

Christos S. Bartsocas, "Two Fourteenth Century Greek Descriptions of the 'Black Death,'"
Journal of the History of Medicine, October 1966.

So incurable was the evil, that neither any regularity of life, nor any bodily strength could resist it. Strong and weak bodies were all similarly carried away, and those best cared for died in the same manner as the poor. No other disease of

---

The Plague in the Muslim World

In his book The Black Death: Natural and Human Disaster in Medieval Europe, *historian Robert Gottfried describes the effects of the plague in the Arab world and quotes the Arab historian Ibn Khaldūn, who witnessed the Black Death firsthand.*

By 1349, the entire Islamic world had been engulfed by the Black Death. About a third of the general population and perhaps 40% to 50% of those living in towns had died. The effect was summed up by Ibn Khaldūn, both of whose parents perished:

> Civilization both in the East and the West was visited by a destructive plague which devastated nations and caused populations to vanish. It swallowed up many of the good things of civilization and wiped them out. It overtook the dynasties at the time of their senility, when they had reached the limit of their duration. It lessened their power and curtailed their influence. It weakened their authority. Their situation approached the point of annihilation and dissolution. Civilization decreased with the decrease of mankind. Cities and buildings were laid waste, roads and way signs were obliterated, settlements and mansions became empty, and dynasties and tribes grew weak. The entire inhabited world changed. The East, it seems, was similarly visited, though in accordance with and in proportion to [the East's more affluent] civilization. It was as if the voice of existence in the world had called out for oblivion and restriction and the world responded to its call. God inherits the earth and whoever is upon it.

Robert S. Gottfried, *The Black Death: Natural and Human Disaster in Medieval Europe.* New York: Free Press, 1983.

any kind presented itself that year. If someone had a previous illness he always succumbed to this disease and no physician's art was sufficient; neither did the disease take the same course in all persons, but the others, unable to resist, died the same day, a few even within the hour. Those who could resist for two or three days had a very violent fever at first, the disease in such cases attacking the head; they suffered from speechlessness and insensibility to all happenings and then appeared as if sunken into a deep sleep. Then, if from time to time they came to themselves, they wanted to speak but the tongue was hard to move and they uttered inarticulate sounds because the nerves around the occiput [head] were dead; and they died suddenly. In others, the evil attacked not the head, but the lung, and forthwith there was inflammation inside which produced very sharp pains in the chest.

Sputum suffused with blood was brought up and disgusting and stinking breath from within. The throat and tongue, parched from the heat, were black and congested with blood. It made no difference if they drank much or little. Sleeplessness and weakness were established forever.

Abscesses formed on the upper and lower arms, in a few also in the maxillae [jaws], and in others on other parts of the body. In some they were large and in others small. Black blisters appeared. Some people broke out with black spots all over their bodies; in some they were few and very manifest; in others they were obscure and dense. Everyone died the same death from these symptoms. In some people all the symptoms appeared, in others more or fewer of them, and in no small number [of cases] even one of these was sufficient to provoke death. Those few who were able to escape from among the many who died, were no longer possessed by the same evil, but were safe. The disease did not attack twice in order to kill them.

Great abscesses were formed on the legs or the arms, from which, when cut, a large quantity of foul-smelling pus flowed and the disease was differentiated as that which discharged much annoying matter. Even many who were seized by all the symptoms unexpectedly recovered. There was no help from anywhere; if someone brought to another a remedy useful to himself, this became poison to the other patient. Some, by treating others, became infected with the disease. It caused great destruction and many homes were deserted by their inhabitants. Domestic animals died together with their masters. Most terrible was the discouragement. Whenever people felt sick there was no hope left for recovery, but by turning to despair, adding to their prostration and severely aggravating their sickness, they died at once. No words could express the nature of the disease. All that can be pointed out is that it had nothing in common with the everyday evils to which the nature of man is subject, but was something else sent by God to restore chastity. Many of the sick turned to better things in their minds, by being chastened, not only those who died, but also those who overcame the disease. They abstained from all vice during that time and they lived virtuously; many divided their property among the poor, even before they were attacked by the disease. If he ever felt himself seized, no one was so ruthless as not to show repentance of his faults and to appear before the judgment seat of God with the best chance of salvation, not believing that the soul was incurable or unhealed. Many died in Byzantium then, and the king's son, Andronikos, was attacked and died the third day.

The Plague Arrives in Europe

Gabriele de Mussis

In the fall of 1347, a small fleet of Genoese ships reached the port of Messina, Sicily. They had sailed from the port of Kaffa, in the Crimean Peninsula on the northern shores of the Black Sea, in flight from a siege by the Tartars, nomadic warriors from eastern Asia who had invaded the lands north of Kaffa (modern-day Russia and Ukraine) in the thirteenth century. At Kaffa, the Tatar armies had deliberately infected their enemies with the plague by catapulting dead bodies over the town walls. Rats and dying sailors aboard the ships then brought the infection to Messina, where hundreds of people began suffering the plague's telltale symptoms. Too late to quarantine the death-dealing vessels, the city authorities banished the ships from the port, an action that soon spread the plague to other towns on Sicily and to the mainland of Italy.

In the following account, Gabriele de Mussis (ca. 1280–1356), a notary of the Italian town of Piacenza, describes the early spread of the plague through the cities and ports of Italy. Using apocalyptic imagery, and imagining the motives and the words of an angry and vengeful God, the author describes the spread of the plague as divine punishment for the sins and corruption of human beings. For centuries, historians believed that de Mussis was an eyewitness to the events he described, but documents unearthed in the late nineteenth century show that de Mussis never left Piacenza. Nevertheless, he was certainly an eyewitness to the horrors of the plague, and the

A.W. Henschel, *Archiv für die Gesammte Medicin*, edited by Heinrich Haeser, II. Jena, 1841.

events that followed were probably recounted to him by individuals who knew of them firsthand.

In the name of God, amen. Here begins an account of the disease or mortality which occured in 1348, put together by Gabriele de' Mussis of Piacenza.

May this stand as a perpetual reminder to everyone, now living and yet to be born, how almighty God, king of heaven, lord of the living and of the dead, who holds all things in his hand, looked down from heaven and saw the entire human race wallowing in the mire of manifold wickedness, enmeshed in wrongdoing, pursuing numberless vices, drowning in a sea of depravity because of a limitless capacity for evil, bereft of all goodness, not fearing the judgements of God, and chasing after everything evil, regardless of how hateful and loathsome it was. Seeing such things he called out to the earth: 'What are you doing, held captive by gangs of worthless men, soiled with the filth of sinners? Are you totally helpless? What are you doing? Why do you not demand human blood in vengeance for this wrongdoing? Why do you tolerate my enemies and adversaries? When confronted by such wantonness you should have swallowed my opponents. Make yourself ready to exercise the vengeance which lies within your power.'

And the earth replied, 'I, established by your power, shall open and swallow up the countless criminals as soon as you give the word. When the enraged Judge gives the signal, with violent thunder from heaven, and leads the elements, the planets, the stars and the orders of angels against the human race in an unspeakable judgement, enlisting all forms of life to wipe out the sinners at one savage stroke, I shall refuse the usual harvest, I shall not yield grain, wine and oil.'

God Vows Punishment for Worldly Sins

God said, 'The exercise of justice belongs to me. I am the life of the living. I bear the keys of death. I bring retribution, giving each individual his due. My hands shaped the heavens. I formed light, created the world and adorned it. Oh you sinner, wretched and yet more wretched, why have you chosen to resist me and to scorn all my commands, laws and judgements? Where is the faith of baptism and the price of my redemption? When I fashioned my creation I never imagined that you would fall into these snares and come to this end. I had prepared heaven for you, not hell, and look where you have brought yourself. When you compelled me, who upheld the spheres, to descend into the womb of a virgin I endured hunger, thirst, toil, crucifixion and death—and your deeds, you ingrate, condemn me still to the cross. I ought to have punished you with eternal death, but pity conquered me. Behold, I have been merciful towards you, and you have barely acknowledged the salvation you have gained through me. You are unworthy of eternal bliss, showing yourself instead to be worthy of the torments of hell. Leave my earth, I abandon you to be torn into pieces by dragons. You shall go into the shadows, where there will be perpetual wailing and gnashing of teeth. Now disaster is at hand; your strength must have an end. The sight of the vanities and lecheries to which you have abandoned yourself has provoked me to fury. May evil spirits arise with the power to devour you. May you have no escape from this time forward.

'I pronounce these judgements: may your joys be turned to mourning, your prosperity be shaken by adversity, the course of your life be passed in never-ending terror. Behold the image of death. Behold I open the infernal floodgates. Let hunger strike down those it seizes; let peace be driven from the ends of the earth; let dissensions arise; let kingdoms be consumed in detestable war; let mercy perish throughout the world; let disasters, plagues, violence, robberies, strife and all kinds of wickedness arise. Next, at my command, let the planets poison the air and corrupt the whole earth; let there be universal grief and lamentation. Let the sharp arrows of sudden death have dominion throughout the world. Let no one be spared, either for their sex or their age; let the innocent perish with the guilty and no one escape.

Vengeance on the Church

'Because those I appointed to be shepherds of the world have behaved towards their flocks like ravening wolves, and do not preach the word of God, but neglect all the Lord's business and have barely even urged repentance, I shall take a savage vengeance on them. I shall wipe them from the face of the earth. The enemy and adversary will seize their hidden treasure. They, along with all other wrongdoers, will bear the heavy burden of their offences. Their office—acquired through deceit—will not avail them, and because they feared men rather than God, and valued their grace more highly, they will be branded as hypocrites. Religion, turned out of doors, will grieve. The treacherous and maleficent fellowship of priests and clergy, imperilled by their own failings, will be destroyed. No one will be given rest, poisoned arrows will strike everyone, fevers will throw down the proud, and incurable disease will strike like lightning.'

After this warning had been given to mortals, disease was sent forth; the quivering spear of the Almighty was aimed everywhere and infected the whole human race with its pitiless wounds. Orion, that cruel star, and the tail of the dragon and the angel hurling vials of poison into the sea, and the appalling weather of Saturn were given leave to harm land and sea, men and trees; advancing from east to west with plague-bearing steps they poured out the poisoned vessels throughout the countries of the world, leaving fiery tokens on the sick. And so the terrible violence of death, running through the world threatening ruin, devoured mortals by a sudden blow, as I shall describe below. Mourn, mourn, you peoples, and call upon the mercy of God.

A Mysterious Sickness in the East

In 1346, in the countries of the East, countless numbers of Tartars and Saracens were struck down by a mysterious illness which brought sudden death. Within these countries broad regions, far-spreading provinces, magnificent kingdoms, cities, towns and settlements, ground down by illness and devoured by dreadful death, were soon stripped of their inhabitants. An eastern settlement under the rule of the Tartars called Tana, which lay to the north of Constantinople and was much frequented by Italian merchants, was totally abandoned after an incident there which led to its being besieged and attacked by hordes of Tartars who gathered in a short space of time. The Christian merchants, who had been driven out by force, were so terrified of the power of the Tartars that, to save themselves and their belongings, they fled in an armed ship to Caffa, a settlement in the same part of the world which had been founded long ago by the Genoese.

Oh God! See how the heathen Tartar races, pouring together from all sides, suddenly invested the city of Caffa and besieged the trapped Christians there for almost three years. There, hemmed in by an immense army, they could hardly draw breath, although food could be shipped in, which offered them some hope. But behold, the whole army was affected by a disease which overran the Tartars and killed thousands upon thousands every day. It was as though arrows were raining down from heaven to strike and crush the Tartars' arrogance. All medical advice and attention was useless; the Tartars died as soon as the signs of disease appeared on their bodies: swellings in the armpit or groin caused by coagulating humours, followed by a putrid fever.

The dying Tartars, stunned and stupefied by the immensity of the disaster brought about by the disease, and realising that they had no hope of escape, lost interest in the siege. But they ordered corpses to be placed in catapults and lobbed into the city in the hope that the intolerable stench would kill everyone inside. What seemed like mountains of dead were thrown into the city, and the Christians could not hide or flee or escape from them, although they dumped as many of the bodies as they could in the sea. And soon the rotting corpses tainted the air and poisoned the water supply, and the stench was so overwhelming that hardly one in several thousand was in a position to flee the remains of the Tartar army. Moreover one infected man could carry the poison to others, and infect people and places with the disease by look alone. No one knew, or could discover, a means of defence.

Thus almost everyone who had been in the East, or in the regions to the south and north, fell victim to sudden death after contracting this pestilential disease, as if struck by a lethal arrow which raised a tumour on their bodies. The scale of the mortality and the form which it took persuaded those who lived, weeping and lamenting, through the bitter events of 1346 to 1348—the Chinese, Indians, Persians, Medes, Kurds, Armenians, Cilicians, Georgians, Mesopotamians, Nubians, Ethiopians, Turks, Egyptians, Arabs, Saracens and Greeks (for almost all the East has been affected)—that the last judgement had come. . . .

The Genoese Bring the Plague to Europe

As it happened, among those who escaped from Caffa by boat were a few sailors who had been infected with the poisonous disease. Some boats were bound for Genoa, others went to Venice and to other Christian areas. When the sailors reached these places and mixed with the people there, it was as if they had brought evil spirits with them: every city, every settlement, every place was poisoned by the contagious pestilence, and their inhabitants, both men and women, died suddenly. And when one person had contracted the illness, he poisoned his whole family even as he fell and died, so that those preparing to bury his body were seized by death in the same way. Thus death entered through the windows, and as cities and towns were depopulated their inhabitants mourned their dead neighbours. . . .

When they returned to their own folk, these people speedily poisoned the whole family, and within three days the afflicted family would succumb to the dart of death. Mass funerals had to be held and there was not enough room to bury the growing numbers of dead. Priests and doctors, upon whom most of the care of the sick devolved, had their hands full in visiting the sick and, alas, by the time they left they too had been infected and followed the dead immediately to the grave. Oh fathers! Oh mothers! Oh children and wives! For a long time prosperity preserved you from harm, but one grave now covers you and the unfortunate alike. You who enjoyed the world and upon whom pleasure and prosperity smiled, who mingled joys with follies, the same tomb receives you and you are handed over as food for worms. Oh hard death, impious death, bitter death, cruel death, who divides parents, divorces spouses, parts children, separates brothers and sisters. We bewail our wretched plight. The past has devoured us, the present is gnawing our entrails, the future threatens yet greater dangers. What we laboured to amass with feverish activity, we have lost in one hour.

Where are the fine clothes of gilded youth? Where is nobility and the courage of fighters, where the mature wisdom of elders and the regal throng of great ladies, where the piles of treasure and precious stones? Alas! All have been destroyed; thrust aside by death. To whom shall we turn, who can help us? To flee is impossible, to hide futile. Cities, fortresses, fields, woods, highways and rivers are ringed by thieves—which is to say by evil spirits, the executioners of the supreme Judge, preparing endless punishments for us all.

We can unfold a terrifying event which happened when an army was camped near Genoa. Four of the soldiers left the force in search of plunder and made their way to Rivarolo on the coast, where the disease had killed all the inhabitants. Finding the houses shut up, and no one about, they broke into one of the houses and stole a fleece which they found on a bed. They then rejoined the army and on the following night the four of them bedded down under the fleece. When morning comes it finds them dead. As a result everyone panicked, and thereafter nobody would use the goods and clothes of the dead, or even handle them, but rejected them outright.

Ravaging Italy and the East

Scarcely one in seven of the Genoese survived. In Venice, where an inquiry was held into the mortality, it was found that more than 70% of the people had died, and that within a short period 20 out of 24 excellent physicians had died. The rest of Italy, Sicily and Apulia and the neighbouring regions maintain that they have been virtually emptied of inhabitants. The people of Florence, Pisa and Lucca, finding themselves bereft of their fellow residents, emphasise their losses. The Roman Curia [papal court] at Avignon, the provinces on both sides of the Rhône, Spain, France, and the [German] Empire cry up their griefs and disasters—all of which makes it extraordinarily difficult for me to give an accurate picture.

By contrast, what befell the Saracens can be established from trustworthy accounts. In the city of Babylon alone (the heart of the Sultan's power), 480,000 of his subjects are said to have been carried off by disease in less than three months in 1348—and this is known from the Sultan's register which records the names of the dead, because he receives a gold bezant for each person buried. I am silent about Damascus and his other cities, where the number of dead was infinite. In the other countries of the East, which are so vast that it takes three years to ride across them and which have a population of 10,000 for every one inhabitant of the west, it is credibly reported that countless people have died.

Plague in Piacenza

Everyone has a responsibility to keep some record of the disease and the deaths, and because I am myself from Piacenza I have been urged to write more about what happened there in 1348. Some Genoese, whom the disease had forced to flee, crossed the Alps in search of a safe place to live and so came to Lombardy. Some had merchandise with them and sold it while they were staying in Bobbio, whereupon the purchaser, their host, and his whole household, together with several neighbours, were infected and died suddenly of the disease. One man there, wanting to make his will, died along with the notary, the priest who heard his confession, and the people summoned to witness the will, and they were all buried together on the following day. The scale of the disaster was such that virtually all the inhabitants were subsequently struck down by sudden death and only a tiny handful remained alive.

Another of the Genoese, who was already suffering from

the illness, managed to reach Piacenza. Finding himself unwell, he sought out his close friend Fulco della Croce, who gave him shelter. He immediately took to his bed and died, and then straightaway Fulco, with his whole household and many of the neighbours, died too. And that, briefly, is how this disease (spreading rapidly throughout the world) arrived in Piacenza. I don't know where to begin. Cries and laments arise on all sides. Day after day one sees the Cross and the Host being carried about the city, and countless dead being buried. The ensuing mortality was so great that people could scarcely snatch breath. The living made preparations for

A Poet's Description of the Black Death

The Welsh poet Jeuan Gethin gave the following account of the plague's arrival in his country in April 1349.

We see death coming into our midst like black smoke, a plague which cuts off the young, a rootless phantom which has no mercy for fair countenance. Woe is me of the shilling in the arm-pit; it is seething, terrible, wherever it may come, a head that gives pain and causes a loud cry, a burden carried under the arms, a painful angry knob, a white lump. It is of the form of an apple, like the head of an onion, a small boil that spares no one. Great is its seething, like a burning cinder, a grievous thing of an ashy colour. It is an ugly eruption that comes with unseemly haste. They are similar to the seeds of the black peas, broken fragments of brittle sea-coal and crowds precede the end. It is a grievous ornament that breaks out in a rash. They are like a shower of peas, the early ornaments of black death, cinders of the peelings of the cockle weed, a mixed multitude, a black plague like halfpence, like berries. It is a grievous thing that they should be on a fair skin.

Philip Ziegler, *The Black Death.* New York: John Day, 1969.

their burial, and because there was not enough room for individual graves, pits had to be dug in colonnades and piazzas, where nobody had ever been buried before. It often happened that man and wife, father and son, mother and daughter, and soon the whole household and many neighbours, were buried together in one place. The same thing happened in Castell' Arquato and Viguzzolo and in the other towns, villages, cities and settlements, and last of all in the Val Tidone, where they had hitherto escaped the plague.

Very many people died. One Oberto de Sasso, who had come from the infected neighbourhood around the church of the Franciscans, wished to make his will and accordingly summoned a notary and his neighbours as witnesses, all of whom, more than sixty of them, died soon after. At this time the Dominican friar Syfredo de Bardis, a man of prudence and great learning who had visited the Holy Sepulchre, also died, along with 23 brothers of the same house. There also died within a short time the Franciscan friar Bertolino Coxadocha of Piacenza, renowned for his learning and many virtues, along with 24 brothers of the same house, nine of them on one day; seven of the Augustinians; the Carmelite friar Francesco Todischi with six of his brethren; four of the order of Mary; more than sixty prelates and parish priests from the city and district of Piacenza; many nobles; countless young people; numberless women, particularly those who were pregnant. It is too distressing to recite any more, or to lay bare the wounds inflicted by so great a disaster.

Taking Pity on the Sick

Let all creation tremble with fear before the judgement of God. Let human frailty submit to its creator. May a greater grief be kindled in all hearts, and tears well up in all eyes as future ages hear what happened in this disaster. When one person lay sick in a house no one would come near. Even dear friends would hide themselves away, weeping. The physician would not visit. The priest, panic-stricken, administered the sacraments with fear and trembling.

Listen to the tearful voices of the sick: 'Have pity, have

pity, my friends. At least say something, now that the hand of God has touched me.'

'Oh father, why have you abandoned me? Do you forget that I am your child?'

'Mother, where have you gone? Why are you now so cruel to me when only yesterday you were so kind? You fed me at your breast and carried me within your womb for nine months.'

'My children, whom I brought up with toil and sweat, why have you run away?'

Man and wife reached out to each other, 'Alas, once we slept happily together but now are separated and wretched.'

And when the sick were in the throes of death, they still called out piteously to their family and neighbours, 'Come here. I'm thirsty, bring me a drink of water. I'm still alive. Don't be frightened. Perhaps I won't die. Please hold me tight, hug my wasted body. You ought to be holding me in your arms.'

At this, as everyone else kept their distance, somebody might take pity and leave a candle burning by the bed head as he fled. And when the victim had breathed his last, it was often the mother who shrouded her son and placed him in the coffin, or the husband who did the same for his wife, for everybody else refused to touch the dead body. No prayer, trumpet or bell summoned friends and neighbours to the funeral, nor was mass performed. Degraded and poverty-striken wretches were paid to carry the great and noble to burial, for the social equals of the dead person dared not attend the funeral for fear of being struck down themselves. Men were borne to burial by day and night, since needs must, and with only a short service. In many cases the houses of the dead had to be shut up, for no one dared enter them or touch the belongings of the dead. No one knew what to do. Everyone, one by one, fell in turn to death's dart.

What a tragic and wretched sight! Who would not shed sympathetic tears? Who would not be shaken by the disastrous plague and the terrors of death? But our hearts have grown hard now that we have no future to look forward to.

Alas. Our inheritance has been diverted to strangers, our homes to outsiders. It is only the survivors who can enjoy the relief of tears.

I am overwhelmed, I can't go on. Everywhere one turns there is death and bitterness to be described. The hand of the Almighty strikes repeatedly, to greater and greater effect. The terrible judgement gains in power as time goes by.

—What shall we do? Kind Jesus, receive the souls of the dead, avert your gaze from our sins and blot out all our iniquities.

Following a Righteous Path

We know that whatever we suffer is the just reward of our sins. Now, therefore, when the Lord is enraged, embrace acts of penance, so that you do not stray from the right path and perish. Let the proud be humbled. Let misers, who withheld alms from the poor, blush for shame. Let the envious become zealous in almsgiving. Let lechers put aside their filthy habits and distinguish themselves in honest living. Let the raging and wrathful restrain themselves from violence. Let gluttons temper their appetites by fasting. Let the slaves of sloth arise and dress themselves in good works. Let adolescents and youths abandon their present delight in following fashion. Let there be good faith and equity among judges, and respect for the law among merchants. Let pettifogging lawyers study and grow wise before they put pen to paper. Let members of religious orders abandon hypocrisy. Let the dignity of prelates be put to better use. Let all of you hurry to set your feet on the way of salvation. And let the overweening vanity of great ladies, which so easily turns into voluptuousness, be bridled. It was against their arrogance that Isaiah inveighed: 'Because the daughters of Sion are haughty, and have walked with stretched out necks and wanton glances of their eyes, and made a noise as they walked with their feet, and moved in a set pace: the Lord will make bald the crown of the head of the daughters of Sion: and the Lord will discover their hair. In that day, the Lord will take away the ornaments of shoes, and little moons: and chains, and necklaces, and bracelets, and bonnets and bodkins, and ornaments of the legs, and tablets, and sweet balls, and earrings: and rings, and jewels hanging on the forehead: and changes of apparel, and short cloaks, and fine linen, and crisping pins: and looking glasses, and lawns and headbands, and fine veils. And instead of a sweet smell, there shall be a stench: and instead of a girdle, a cord. And instead of curled hair, baldness: and instead of a stomacher, haircloth. Thy fairest men also shall fall by the sword: and thy valiant ones in battle. And her gates shall lament and mourn: and she shall sit desolate on the ground' [Isaiah 3.16–26]. This was directed against the pride of ladies and young people.

Symptoms of the Plague

For the rest, so that the conditions, causes and symptoms of this pestilential disease, should be made plain to all, I have decided to set them out in writing. Those of both sexes who were in health, and in no fear of death, were struck by four savage blows to the flesh. First, out of the blue, a kind of chilly stiffness troubled their bodies. They felt a tingling sensation, as if they were being pricked by the points of arrows. The next stage was a fearsome attack which took the form of an extremely hard, solid boil. In some people this developed under the armpit and in others in the groin between the scrotum and the body. As it grew more solid, its burning heat caused the patients to fall into an acute and putrid fever, with severe headaches. As it intensified its extreme bitterness could have various effects. In some cases it gave rise to an intolerable stench. In others it brought vomiting of blood, or swellings near the place from which the corrupt humour arose: on the back, across the chest, near the thigh. Some people lay as if in a drunken stupor and could not be roused. Behold the swellings, the warning signs sent by the Lord. All these people were in danger of dying. Some died on the very day the illness took possession of them, others on the next day, others—the majority—between the third and fifth day. There was no known remedy for the vomiting of blood.

Those who fell into a coma, or suffered a swelling or the stink of corruption very rarely escaped. But from the fever it was sometimes possible to make a recovery.

I have, however, known a case where, although there was a stench arising from the patient, the use of the best theriac [ointment] expelled the poison and prevented it proving fatal. If the tumid humour revealed itself in numbness, but not by any external growths, it was a sign of death, because then the poison, passing into the veins of the heart, smothered the patient. But if swellings appeared externally, on the upper or lower body, the patient might be rescued. He could be cured by immediately letting blood from the appropriate part of his body: from his arm if the upper part of the body was affected; from the tendon of the foot if it was the lower part which was affected. When this was followed up with medicinal means, using mallow or a plaster of marsh mallow to ripen the boil and draw the humours from the seat of the illness, and then cutting out the boil, the patients received the blessing of health. But if the bitter fever persisted it stole the life of its victims. It can be asserted, on the clear evidence of experience, that the illness was more dangerous during an eclipse, because then its effect was enhanced, and it was at such times that people died in the greatest numbers.

Signs, Visions, and Portents

In the East, in Cathay, which is the greatest country in the world, horrible and terrifying signs appeared. Serpents and toads fell in a thick rain, entered dwellings and devoured numberless people, injecting them with poison and gnawing them with their teeth. In the South, in the Indies, earthquakes cast down whole towns and cities were consumed by fire from heaven. The hot fumes of the fire burnt up infinite numbers of people, and in some places it rained blood, and stones fell from the sky.

Truly, then was a time of bitterness and grief, which served to turn men to the Lord. I shall recount what happened. A warning was given by a certain holy person, who received it in a vision, that in cities, towns and other settlements, everyone, male and female alike, should gather in their parish church on three consecutive days and, each with a lighted candle in their hand, hear with great devotion the mass of the Blessed Anastasia, which is normally performed at dawn on Christmas day, and they should humbly beg for mercy, so that they might be delivered from the disease through the merits of the holy mass. Other people sought deliverance through the mediation of a blessed martyr; and others humbly turned to other saints, so that they might escape the abomination of disease. For among the aforesaid martyrs, some, as stories relate, are said to have died from repeated blows, and it was therefore the general opinion that they would be able to protect people against the arrows of death. Finally, in 1350, the most holy Pope Clement ordained a general indulgence [an official forgiveness of sin], to be valid for a year, which remitted penance and guilt to all who were truly penitent and confessed. And as a result a numberless multitude of people made the pilgrimage to Rome, to visit with great reverence and devotion the basilicas of the blessed apostles Peter and Paul and St John.

Oh, most dearly beloved, let us therefore not be like vipers, growing ever more wicked, but let us rather hold up our hands to heaven to beg for mercy on us all, for who but God shall have mercy on us? With this, I make an end. May the heavenly physician heal our wounds—our spiritual rather than our bodily wounds. To whom be the blessing and the praise and the glory for ever and ever, Amen.

The Great Fear of Florence

Marchione di Coppo Stefani

In his *Florentine Chronicle* (*Cronaca fiorentina*), written in the late 1370s and early 1380s, the Italian chronicler Marchione di Coppo Stefani describes the plague as it struck the city of Florence. Although he was still a teenager at the time the Black Death arrived, Stefani retained vivid memories of the plague's symptoms and how fear of the disease prompted families to abandon their sick loved ones. He also writes of the burial of the plague's victims, who died in such numbers that the survivors forgot ordinary funeral ceremonies and had to dig mass graves for the bodies.

In addition to recording the human toll, Stefani reflects on the economic impact of the plague, which gave rise to an entire class of "vultures," who greatly profited from services they rendered to the dead and dying.

In the year of the Lord 1348 there was a very great pestilence in the city and district of Florence. It was of such a fury and so tempestuous that in houses in which it took hold previously healthy servants who took care of the ill died of the same illness. Almost none of the ill survived past the fourth day. Neither physicians nor medicines were effective. Whether because these illnesses were previously unknown or because physicians had not previously studied them, there seemed to be no cure. There was such a fear that no one seemed to know what to do. When it took hold in a house it

Marchione di Coppo Stefani, "Cronaca Fiorentina," *Rerum Italicarum Scriptores*, vol. 30, edited by Niccolo Rodolico. Citta di Castello: 1903–1913.

often happened that no one remained who had not died. And it was not just that men and women died, but even sentient animals died. Dogs, cats, chickens, oxen, donkeys [and] sheep showed the same symptoms and died of the same disease. And almost none, or very few, who showed these symptoms, were cured.

The symptoms were the following: a bubo [tumor] in the groin, where the thigh meets the trunk; or a small swelling under the armpit; sudden fever; spitting blood and saliva (and no one who spit blood survived it). It was such a frightful thing that when it got into a house, as was said, no one remained. Frightened people abandoned the house and fled to another. Those in town fled to villages. Physicians could not be found because they had died like the others. And those who could be found wanted vast sums in hand before they entered the house. And when they did enter, they checked the pulse with face turned away. They inspected the urine from a distance and with something odoriferous under their nose. Child abandoned the father, husband the wife, wife the husband, one brother the other, one sister the other. In all the city there was nothing to do but to carry the dead to a burial. And those who died had neither confessor nor other sacraments. And many died with no one looking after them. And many died of hunger because when someone took to bed sick, another in the house, terrified, said to him: "I'm going for the doctor." Calmly walking out the door, the other left and did not return again.

Abandoned by people, without food, but accompanied by fever, they weakened. There were many who pleaded with their relatives not to abandon them when night fell. But [the relatives] said to the sick person, "So that during the night you did not have to awaken those who serve you and who work hard day and night, take some sweetmeats, wine or water. They are here on the bedstead by your head; here are some blankets." And when the sick person had fallen asleep, they left and did not return. If it happened that he was strengthened by the food during the night he might be alive and strong enough to get to the window. If the street was not a major one, he might stand there a half hour before anyone came by. And if someone did pass by, and if he was strong enough that he could be heard when he called out to them, sometimes there might be a response and sometimes not, but there was no help. No one, or few, wished to enter a house where anyone was sick, nor did they even want to deal with those healthy people who came out of a sick person's house. And they said to them: "He is stupefied, do not speak to him!" saying further: "He has it because there is a bubo in his house." They call the swelling a bubo.

Many died unseen. So they remained in their beds until they stank. And the neighbors, if there were any, having smelled the stench, placed them in a shroud and sent them for burial. The house remained open and yet there was no one daring enough to touch anything because it seemed that things remained poisoned and that whoever used them picked up the illness.

At every church, or at most of them, they dug deep trenches, down to the waterline, wide and deep, depending on how large the parish was. And those who were responsible for the dead carried them on their backs in the night in which they died and threw them into the ditch, or else they paid a high price to those who would do it for them. The next morning, if there were many [bodies] in the trench, they covered them over with dirt. And then more bodies were put on top of them, with a little more dirt over those; they put layer on layer just like one puts layers of cheese in a lasagna.

The beccamorti [literally, "vultures"] who provided their service, were paid such a high price that many were enriched by it. Many died from [carrying away the dead], some rich, some after earning just a little, but high prices continued. Servants, or those who took care of the ill, charged from one to three florins per day and the cost of things grew. The things that the sick ate, sweetmeats and sugar, seemed priceless. Sugar cost from three to eight florins per pound. And other confections cost similarly. Capons and other poultry were very expensive and eggs cost between twelve and twenty-four pence each; and he was blessed who could find three per day even if he searched the entire city. Finding wax was miraculous. A pound of wax would have gone up more than a florin if there had not been a stop put [by the communal government] to the vain ostentation that the Florentines always make [over funerals]. Thus it was ordered that no more than two large candles could be carried [in any funeral]. Churches had no more than a single bier which usually was not sufficient. Spice dealers and beccamorti sold biers, burial palls, and cushions at very high prices. Dressing in expensive woolen cloth as is customary in [mourning] the dead, that is in a long cloak, with mantle and veil that used to cost women three florins climbed in price to thirty florins and would have climbed to 100 florins had the custom of dressing in expensive cloth not been changed. The rich dressed in modest woolens, those not rich sewed [clothes] in linen. Benches on which the dead were placed cost like the heavens and still the benches were only a hundredth of those needed.

Priests were not able to ring bells as they would have liked. Concerning that [the government] issued ordinances discouraging the sounding of bells, sale of burial benches, and limiting expenses. They could not sound bells, sell benches, nor cry out announcements because the sick hated to hear of this and it discouraged the healthy as well. Priests and friars went [to serve] the rich in great multitudes and they were paid such high prices that they all got rich. And therefore [the authorities] ordered that one could not have more than a prescribed number [of clerics] of the local parish church. And the prescribed number of friars was six. All fruits with a nut at the center, like unripe plums and unhusked almonds, fresh broadbeans, figs and every useless and unhealthy fruit, were forbidden entrance into the city. Many processions, including those with relics and the painted tablet of Santa Maria Inpruneta, went through the city crying our "Mercy" and praying and then they came to a stop in the piazza of the Priors. There they made peace concerning important controversies, injuries and deaths.

This [pestilence] was a matter of such great discouragement and fear that men gathered together in order to take some comfort in dining together. And each evening one of them provided dinner to ten companions and the next evening they planned to eat with one of the others. And sometimes if they planned to eat with a certain one he had no meal prepared because he was sick. Or if the host had made dinner for the ten, two or three were missing. Some fled to villas, others to villages in order to get a change of air. Where there had been no [pestilence], there they carried it; if it was already there, they caused it to increase. None of the guilds [craft associations] in Florence was working. All the shops were shut, taverns closed; only the apothecaries and the churches remained open. If you went outside, you found almost no one. And many good and rich men were carried from home to church on a pall by four beccamorti and one tonsured clerk who carried the cross. Each of them wanted a florin. This mortality enriched apothecaries [drugists], doctors, poultry vendors, beccamorti, and green-grocers who sold of poultices of mallow [an herb], nettles, mercury and other herbs necessary to draw off the infirmity. And it was those who made these poultices who made a lot of money. Woolworkers and vendors of remnants of cloth who found themselves in possession of cloths [after the death of the entrepreneur for whom they were working] sold it to whoever asked for it. When the mortality ended, those who found themselves with cloth of any kind or with raw materials for making cloth was enriched. But many [who actually owned cloths being processed by workers] found it to be moth-eaten, ruined or lost by the weavers. Large quantities of raw and processed wool were lost throughout the city and countryside.

This pestilence began in March, as was said, and ended in September 1348. And people began to return to look after their houses and possessions. And there were so many houses full of goods without a master that it was stupefying. Then those who would inherit these goods began to appear. And such it was that those who had nothing found themselves rich with what did not seem to be theirs and they were unseemly because of it. Women and men began to dress ostentatiously. . . .

Economic Effects of the Plague in Florence

In the said year, when the mortality stopped, women and men in Florence were unmindful of [traditional modesty concerning] their dress. And ordinances were passed concerning this giving authority to the Judge of the Grascia to enforce these ordinances. The tailors made such boundless demands for payment that they could not be satisfied. Authority was granted [to the judge] that he should handle all matters himself. Servants were so unhappy about the very high prices [they paid] that it was necessary to make great efforts to restrain [the price rises]. The workers on the land in the countryside wanted rent contracts such that you could say that all they harvested would be theirs. And they learned to demand oxen from the landlord but at the landlord's risk [and liability for any harm done to the animal]. And then they helped others for pay by the job or by the day. And they also learned to deny [liability for] loans and [rental] payments. Concerning this serious ordinances were instituted; and [hiring] laborers became much more expensive. You could say that the farms were theirs; and they wanted the oxen, seed, loans quickly and on good terms. It was necessary to put a brake on weddings as well because when they gathered for the betrothal each party brought too many people in order to increase the pomp. And thus the wedding was made up of so many trappings. How many days were necessary and how many women took part in a woman's wedding. And they passed many other ordinances concerning [these issues].

Escaping the Black Death

Giovanni Boccaccio

> *The Decameron* of Giovanni Boccaccio, who lived from 1313
> to 1375, has become one of the best-known works of
> medieval literature. According to the author, this collection of
> one hundred stories was recounted by a group of ten young
> men and women who sought refuge from the plague in a
> country house. In his introduction to *The Decameron*, which
> is excerpted here, Boccaccio created a graphic and disturbing
> description of the plague that became, through the fame of
> the book that follows, the best-known contemporary account
> of the Black Death.
>
> Although *The Decameron* is fictional, the setting of the
> book and the circumstances described in the introduction
> were all too real. Nevertheless, historians have long debated
> whether Boccaccio himself was ever present in the city of
> Florence during the Black Death. If not, he was given details
> of the sickness from friends and from his father, a banker who
> was serving the city government at the time as the master of
> supply. Shortly after the plague's arrival in Florence, Boccac-
> cio's father died. Assuming a new role as head of his family,
> Boccaccio left his cloistered life as a scholar and began work
> on *The Decameron*.

I say, then, that the sum of thirteen hundred and forty-eight
years had elapsed since the fruitful Incarnation of the
Son of God, when the noble city of Florence, which for its

great beauty excels all others in Italy, was visited by the deadly pestilence. Some say that it descended upon the human race through the influence of the heavenly bodies, others that it was a punishment signifying God's righteous anger at our iniquitous way of life. But whatever its cause, it had originated some years earlier in the East, where it had claimed countless lives before it unhappily spread westward, growing in strength as it swept relentlessly on from one place to the next.

In the face of its onrush, all the wisdom and ingenuity of man were unavailing. Large quantities of refuse were cleared out of the city by officials specially appointed for the purpose, all sick persons were forbidden entry, and numerous instructions were issued for safeguarding the people's health, but all to no avail. Nor were the countless petitions humbly directed to God by the pious, whether by means of formal processions or in all other ways, any less ineffectual. For in the early spring of the year we have mentioned, the plague began, in a terrifying and extraordinary manner, to make its disastrous effects apparent. It did not take the form it had assumed in the East, where if anyone bled from the nose it was an obvious portent of certain death. On the contrary, its earliest symptom, in men and women alike, was the appearance of certain swellings in the groin or the armpit, some of which were eggshaped whilst others were roughly the size of the common apple. Sometimes the swellings were large, sometimes not so large, and they were referred to by the populace as *gavòccioli*. From the two areas already mentioned, this deadly *gavòcciolo* would begin to spread, and within a short time it would appear at random all over the body. Later on, the symptoms of the disease changed, and many people began to find dark blotches and bruises on their arms, thighs, and other parts of the body, sometimes large and few in number, at other times tiny and closely spaced. These, to anyone unfortunate enough to contract them, were just as infallible a sign that he would die as the *gavòcciolo* had been earlier, and as indeed it still was.

Against these maladies, it seemed that all the advice of physicians and all the power of medicine were profitless and unavailing. Perhaps the nature of the illness was such that it allowed no remedy: or perhaps those people who were treating the illness (whose numbers had increased enormously because the ranks of the qualified were invaded by people, both men and women, who had never received any training in medicine), being ignorant of its causes, were not prescribing the appropriate cure. At all events, few of those who caught it ever recovered, and in most cases death occurred within three days from the appearance of the symptoms we have described, some people dying more rapidly than others, the majority without any fever or other complications.

The Rapid Spread of the Plague

But what made this pestilence even more severe was that whenever those suffering from it mixed with people who were still unaffected, it would rush upon these with the speed of a fire racing through dry or oily substances that happened to come within its reach. Nor was this the full extent of its evil, for not only did it infect healthy persons who conversed or had any dealings with the sick, making them ill or visiting an equally horrible death upon them, but it also seemed to transfer the sickness to anyone touching the clothes or other objects which had been handled or used by its victims.

It is a remarkable story that I have to relate. And were it not for the fact that I am one of many people who saw it with their own eyes, I would scarcely dare to believe it, let alone commit it to paper, even though I had heard it from a person whose word I could trust. The plague I have been describing was of so contagious a nature that very often it visibly did more than simply pass from one person to another. In other words, whenever an animal other than a human being touched anything belonging to a person who had been stricken or exterminated by the disease, it not only caught the sickness, but died from it almost at once. To all of this, as I have just said, my own eyes bore witness on more than one occasion. One day, for instance, the rags of a pauper who had died from the disease were thrown into the street, where they attracted the attention of two pigs. In their wonted fashion, the pigs first of all gave the rags a thorough mauling with their snouts, after which they took them between their teeth and shook them against their cheeks. And within a short time they began to writhe as though they had been poisoned, then they both dropped dead to the ground, spread-eagled upon the rags that had brought about their undoing.

These things, and many others of a similar or even worse nature, caused various fears and fantasies to take root in the minds of those who were still alive and well. And almost without exception, they took a single and very inhuman precaution, namely to avoid or run away from the sick and their belongings, by which means they all thought that their own health would be preserved.

Trying to Escape the Plague

Some people were of the opinion that a sober and abstemious mode of living considerably reduced the risk of infection. They therefore formed themselves into groups and lived in isolation from everyone else. Having withdrawn to a comfortable abode where there were no sick persons, they locked themselves in and settled down to a peaceable existence, consuming modest quantities of delicate foods and precious wines and avoiding all excesses. They refrained from speaking to outsiders, refused to receive news of the dead or the sick, and entertained themselves with music and whatever other amusements they were able to devise.

Others took the opposite view, and maintained that an infallible way of warding off this appalling evil was to drink heavily, enjoy life to the full, go round singing and merrymaking, gratify all of one's cravings whenever the opportunity offered, and shrug the whole thing off as one enormous joke. Moreover, they practised what they preached to the best of their ability, for they would visit one tavern after another, drinking all day and night to immoderate excess; or alternatively (and this was their more frequent custom), they would do their drinking in various private houses, but only in the ones where the conversation was restricted to subjects that were pleasant or entertaining. Such places were easy to find, for people behaved as though their days were numbered, and treated their belongings and their own persons with equal abandon. Hence most houses had become common property, and any passing stranger could make himself at home as naturally as though he were the rightful owner. But for all their riotous manner of living, these people always took good care to avoid any contact with the sick.

In the face of so much affliction and misery, all respect for the laws of God and man had virtually broken down and been extinguished in our city. For like everybody else, those ministers and executors of the laws who were not either dead or ill were left with so few subordinates that they were unable to discharge any of their duties. Hence everyone was free to behave as he pleased.

There were many other people who steered a middle course between the two already mentioned, neither restricting their diet to the same degree as the first group, nor indulging so freely as the second in drinking and other forms of wantonness, but simply doing no more than satisfy their appetite. Instead of incarcerating themselves, these people moved about freely, holding in their hands a posy of flowers, or fragrant herbs, or one of a wide range of spices, which they applied at frequent intervals to their nostrils, thinking it an excellent idea to fortify the brain with smells of that particular sort; for the stench of dead bodies, sickness, and medicines seemed to fill and pollute the whole of the atmosphere.

Some people, pursuing what was possibly the safer alternative, callously maintained that there was no better or more efficacious remedy against a plague than to run away from it. Swayed by this argument, and sparing no thought for anyone but themselves, large numbers of men and women abandoned their city, their homes, their relatives, their estates and their belongings, and headed for the countryside, either in Florentine territory or, better still, abroad. It was as though they imagined that the wrath of God would not unleash this plague against men for their iniquities irrespective of where they happened to be, but would only be aroused against those who found themselves within the city walls; or possibly they assumed that the whole of the population would be exterminated and that the city's last hour had come.

The Healthy Abandon the Sick

Of the people who held these various opinions, not all of them died. Nor, however, did they all survive. On the contrary, many of each different persuasion fell ill here, there, and everywhere, and having themselves, when they were fit and well, set an example to those who were as yet unaffected, they languished away with virtually no one to nurse them. It was not merely a question of one citizen avoiding another, and of people almost invariably neglecting their neighbours and rarely or never visiting their relatives, ad-

---

Boccaccio's Literary Symptoms

Author of the best-known description of the Black Death, Giovanni Boccaccio escaped the disease but also underwent an important transformation in the wake of the plague, as described by author Robert Gottfried in his book The Black Death: Natural and Human Disaster in Medieval Europe.

As in the fine arts, the Black Death brought changes in literary styles and ideas, most of which were somber. A good example is the later works of Boccaccio. *The Decameron*, his literary masterpiece, was written in the vernacular and was enormously popular. Its cynicism reflected a common perception during and immediately after the Black Death. But his attitudes soon changed. While *The Decameron* is guilt-free, Boccaccio's later works show a more sober side. *The Corbaccio*, written in 1354–55, is gloomy, pessimistic, truculent, and ascetic, attitudes that hardened even more as Boccaccio grew older and began to think about his own salvation. In a 1373 letter, he condemned his earlier masterpiece:

dressing them only from a distance; this scourge had implanted so great a terror in the hearts of men and women that brothers abandoned brothers, uncles their nephews, sisters their brothers, and in many cases wives deserted their husbands. But even worse, and almost incredible, was the fact that fathers and mothers refused to nurse and assist their own children, as though they did not belong to them.

Hence the countless numbers of people who fell ill, both male and female, were entirely dependent upon either the charity of friends (who were few and far between) or the greed of servants, who remained in short supply despite the attraction of high wages out of all proportion to the services they performed. Furthermore, these latter were men and women of coarse intellect and the majority were unused to such duties, and they did little more than hand things to the invalid when asked to do so and watch over him when he was dying. And in performing this kind of service, they fre-

---

I am certainly not pleased that you have allowed the illustrious women in your house to read my trifles; indeed, I beg you to give me your word that you will not permit it. You know how much in them is less than decent and opposed to modesty, how much stimulation to wanton lust, how many things that drive to lust even those most fortified against it. . . . My feminine readers will judge me a filthy pimp and an incestuous old man, shameless, foul-mouthed and malignant, eager to spread tales of the dissolution of others.

Boccaccio turned against love, passion, and even women; indeed, he became something of a misogynist. Perhaps he was affected by his idol and master, Petrarch. Petrarch lost his beloved Laura and four other intimates to the plague, resigned himself to religion, and turned to introspection. In a letter to Boccaccio, probably from 1363, Petrarch wrote: "Of all my friends, only you remain."

Robert S. Gottfried, *The Black Death: Natural and Human Disaster in Medieval Europe.* New York: Free Press, 1983.

quently lost their lives as well as their earnings.

As a result of this wholesale desertion of the sick by neighbours, relatives and friends, and in view of the scarcity of servants, there grew up a practice almost never previously

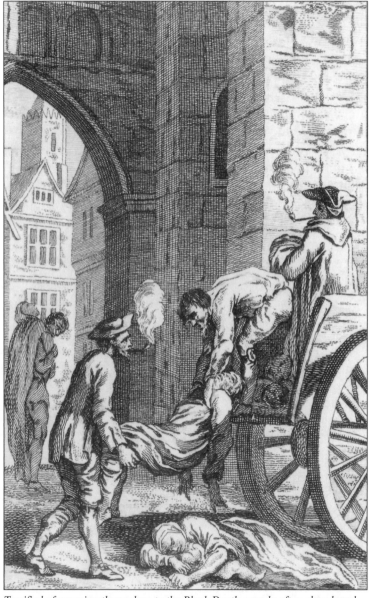

Terrified of exposing themselves to the Black Death, people often abandoned the bodies of dead plague victims in the street.

heard of, whereby when a woman fell ill, no matter how gracious or beautiful or gently bred she might be, she raised no objection to being attended by a male servant, whether he was young or not. Nor did she have any scruples about showing him every part of her body as freely as she would have displayed it to a woman, provided that the nature of her infirmity required her to do so; and this explains why those women who recovered were possibly less chaste in the period that followed.

New Customs

Moreover a great many people died who would perhaps have survived had they received some assistance. And hence, what with the lack of appropriate means for tending the sick, and the virulence of the plague, the number of deaths reported in the city whether by day or by night was so enormous that it astonished all who heard tell of it, to say nothing of the people who actually witnessed the carnage. And it was perhaps inevitable that among the citizens who survived there arose certain customs that were quite contrary to established tradition.

It had once been customary, as it is again nowadays, for the women relatives and neighbours of a dead man to assemble in his house in order to mourn in the company of the women who had been closest to him; moreover his kinsfolk would forgather in front of his house along with his neighbours and various other citizens, and there would be a contingent of priests, whose numbers varied according to the quality of the deceased; his body would be taken thence to the church in which he had wanted to be buried, being borne on the shoulders of his peers amidst the funeral pomp of candles and dirges. But as the ferocity of the plague began to mount, this practice all but disappeared entirely and was replaced by different customs. For not only did people die without having many women about them, but a great number departed this life without anyone at all to witness their going. Few indeed were those to whom the lamentations and bitter tears of their relatives were accorded; on the contrary, more often than not bereavement was the signal for laughter and witticisms and general jollification—the art of which the women, having for the most part suppressed their feminine concern for the salvation of the souls of the dead, had learned to perfection. Moreover it was rare for the bodies of the dead to be accompanied by more than ten or twelve neighbours to the church, nor were they borne on the shoulders of worthy and honest citizens, but by a kind of gravedigging fraternity, newly come into being and drawn from the lower orders of society. These people assumed the title of sexton, and demanded a fat fee for their services, which consisted in taking up the coffin and hauling it swiftly away, not to the church specified by the dead man in his will, but usually to the nearest at hand. They would be preceded by a group of four or six clerics, who between them carried one or two candles at most, and sometimes none at all. Nor did the priests go to the trouble of pronouncing solemn and lengthy funeral rites, but, with the aid of these so-called sextons, they hastily lowered the body into the nearest empty grave they could find.

As for the common people and a large proportion of the bourgeoisie, they presented a much more pathetic spectacle, for the majority of them were constrained, either by their poverty or the hope of survival, to remain in their houses. Being confined to their own parts of the city, they fell ill daily in their thousands, and since they had no one to assist them or attend to their needs, they inevitably perished almost without exception. Many dropped dead in the open streets, both by day and by night, whilst a great many others, though dying in their own houses, drew their neighbours' attention to the fact more by the smell of their rotting corpses than by any other means. And what with these, and the others who were dying all over the city, bodies were here, there and everywhere.

Whenever people died, their neighbours nearly always followed a single, set routine, prompted as much by their fear of being contaminated by the decaying corpse as by any charitable feelings they may have entertained towards the deceased. Either on their own, or with the assistance of bearers whenever these were to be had, they extracted the bodies of the dead from their houses and left them lying outside their front doors, where anyone going about the streets, especially in the early morning, could have observed countless numbers of them. Funeral biers would then be sent for, upon which the dead were taken away, though there were some who, for lack of biers, were carried off on plain boards. It was by no means rare for more than one of these biers to be seen with two or three bodies upon it at a time; on the contrary, many were seen to contain a husband and wife, two or three brothers and sisters, a father and son, or some other pair of close relatives. And times without number it happened that two priests would be on their way to bury someone, holding a cross before them, only to find that bearers carrying three or four additional biers would fall in behind them; so that whereas the priests had thought they had only one burial to attend to, they in fact had six or seven, and sometimes more. Even in these circumstances, however, there were no tears or candles or mourners to honour the dead; in fact, no more respect was accorded to dead people than would nowadays be shown towards dead goats. For it was quite apparent that the one thing which, in normal times, no wise man had ever learned to accept with patient resignation (even though it struck so seldom and unobtrusively), had now been brought home to the feeble-minded as well, but the scale of the calamity caused them to regard it with indifference.

Such was the multitude of corpses (of which further consignments were arriving every day and almost by the hour at each of the churches), that there was not sufficient consecrated ground for them to be buried in, especially if each was to have its own plot in accordance with long-established custom. So when all the graves were full, huge trenches were excavated in the churchyards, into which new arrivals were placed in their hundreds, stowed tier upon tier like ships' cargo, each layer of corpses being covered over with a thin layer of soil till the trench was filled to the top.

A Poet's Agony

Francesco Petrarca

> Among the people of Europe, the Black Death spread a deep fear—a fear so great that it overcame nearly all ties of loyalty to family, friends, and nation. It brought an agonizing questioning of social norms, but it also inspired the poets and chroniclers of the time to set down very moving expressions of their experiences and emotions.
>
> In the flowery poetic language of the following letter to a companion nicknamed Socrates, the Italian writer Francesco Petrarca, known commonly as Petrarch, expresses the anguished soul searching of those who experienced the Black Death. Petrarch, who survived the plague in the city of Parma, had lost not only family and friends but had also suffered the death of Laura. This mysterious woman, whom he had long admired from afar and who inspired his poetry and other writings, died of the Black Death on Good Friday, 1348, in the city of Avignon.

Oh brother, brother, brother (a new kind of beginning for a letter, indeed an ancient one used by Marcus Tullius almost fourteen hundred years ago); alas dearest brother, what shall I say? Where shall I begin? Where shall I turn? Everywhere we see sorrow, on all sides we see terror. In me alone you may see what you read in Virgil concerning so great a city, for "on all sides there is cruel mourning, everywhere there is trembling and countless images of death." Dear brother, would that I had never been born or had died earlier! If I am compelled to wish this now, what do you

Francesco Petrarca, *Rerum Familiarium Libri*, translated by Aldo S. Bernardo. New York: State University of New York Press, 1975. Copyright © 1975 by State University of New York Press. Reproduced by permission.

think I would be saying if I had arrived at a truly old age? Oh would that I never reach that point. But I feel I shall, not because I shall live longer, but because I shall suffer a longer death. Indeed I know my destiny and I slowly understand what I am heading for in this troublesome and unhappy life. Alas, dear brother! I am deeply troubled from within and take pity on myself. What would anyone who hears these words say? "You who seem to offer comfort and aid to others, who had promised us things that were superior, who ought to have formed a thick skin from your constant misfortunes and to have become calloused against all the blows of fortune and hardened to something like a flintstone, see how weakly you bear your burdens, see how often you direct your frequent wailings to us. Where is that loftiness of soul which now especially should mark your profession? Where are the magnificent words, which, if intended rather to extol your genius than as advice for life, can be no more than empty sounds and curious charms for the ears? We expected from you a heroic poem, we get elegiac verses; we hoped for biographies of illustrious heroes, we are getting the story of your sorrow. What we considered letters are laments, where we sought ingenious combinations of words, new molds for language, and sweetly ordered rhetorical colors, we behold nothing but mournful exclamations and indignant tones and tear stains. And what will be the limit or the end if you want to deplore the fate of all mortals? One heart and one tongue would not suffice. Wretched man, you have undertaken a huge and troublesome task which is useless and implacable. You must seek another source for your tears; the recent and continually new causes of grief make it impossible for excessively tired, exhausted, and dried-up eyes to produce sufficient tears. Therefore, forgetful of yourself and dissatisfied with your own misery and illness which you incurred knowingly and willingly, what else are you doing but offering poison to your friends to whom you had promised a cure? Better that you should either cry alone or learn to bear mortal things with the equanimity of a mortal; and noting that not only you or your friends alone, but all living beings are being snatched away, it is time that you put an end to your useless complaining." There may be someone of quick temper who hates such gloomy recitals and will discard them or trample on them with biting scorn saying, "Go to the devil; if you are going to behave like a woman, at least do not prevent us from acting like men." I feel all of these things and none escapes me, dear brother. I realize that a man must either drive away grief or destroy it, or control it, or finally conceal it. But what can I do? I shall die if I cannot pour out my grief in tears and words. My one consolation is that whatever I shall have written, though weak and empty, will reach your hands not as if to a stranger's but as if to my own. Therefore I shall fear no greater shame while you read these things than I felt while I was writing them.

The Storm and Thunder of Fortune

I shall not deny that I did feel some shame; for without the control of reason I felt my mind and my style pulled along with my feelings beyond what I intended, something I find most disturbing. But what I feel to be an even greater insult is that for a whole year and considerably more I have had little occasion, not, indeed, to do, but certainly to write anything worthy of a man as a result of fortune's thundering and storming on all sides. Because of this I may perhaps be excused by a benign judge if he were also to consider that I am bewailing not something inconsequential, but the 1348th year of the sixth age, which not only deprived us of our friends but the entire world of actual nations. If anyone escaped, the coming year is gathering its harvest so that whatever survived that storm is being pursued by death's sickle. How can posterity believe that there was once a time without floods, without fire either from heaven or from earth, without wars, or other visible disaster, in which not only this part or that part of the world, but almost all of it remained without a dweller? When was anything similar either seen or heard? In what chronicles did anyone ever read that dwellings were emptied, cities abandoned, countrysides

filthy, fields laden with bodies, and a dreadful and vast soli-
tude covered the earth? Consult the historians: they are
silent; question the scientists: they are stupified; ask the

The Plague Touches the Rich and Famous

*Although the poor and working classes of Europe were dev-
astated by the Black Death, the epidemic touched all levels
of medieval society. In "A Distant Mirror," her well-known
history of the troubled fourteenth century, Barbara Tuchman gives a short list of the plague's better-known victims.*

Though the death rate was higher among the anonymous
poor, the known and the great died too. King Alfonso
XI of Castile was the only reigning monarch killed by the
pest, but his neighbor King Pedro of Aragon lost his wife,
Queen Leonora, his daughter Marie, and a niece in the
space of six months. . . . In France the lame Queen Jeanne
and her daughter-in-law Bonne de Luxemburg, wife of the
Dauphin, both died in 1349. . . . Jeanne, Queen of Navarre,
daughter of [the French king] Louis X, was another victim.
[The English king] Edward III's second daughter Joanna,
who was on her way to marry Pedro, the heir of Castile,
died in Bordeaux. . . . [The Italian writer Giovanni] Boccaccio's mistress Fiammetta, illegitimate daughter of the
King of Naples, died, as did Lara, the beloved—whether
real or fictional—of [the Italian poet] Petrarch. . . .

In Florence Giovanni Villani, the great historian of his
time, died at 68 in the midst of an unfinished sentence:
". . . *e dure questo pistolenza fino a* . . . (in the midst of the
pestilence there came to an end . . .)." Siena's master
painters, the brothers Ambrogio and Pietro Lorenzetti,
whose names never appear after 1348, presumably perished in the plague, as did Andrea Pisano, architect and
sculptor of Florence. William of Ockham and the English
mystic Richard Rolle of Hampole both disappear from
mention after 1349.

Barbara Tuchman, *A Distant Mirror: The Calamitous Fourteenth Century.* New
York: Alfred A. Knopf, 1978.

philosophers: they shrug their shoulders, they wrinkle their brows and they order silence by holding their fingers to their lips. Will you believe such things, oh posterity, when we ourselves who see them can scarcely believe them and would consider them dreams except that we perceive them awake and with our eyes open and that after viewing a city full of funerals we return to our homes only to find them empty of our loved ones. Should we not indeed know that what we grieve over is indeed true? Oh happy generation of our great-grandsons who will not have known these miseries and perhaps will consider our testimony as fable!

I do not deny that we deserve these things and even worse; but our ancestors also deserved them, and would that our descendants will not! Why is it, then, oh most blessed judge, why is it that the violence of your vengeance lies so extraordinary upon our times? Why is it that when guilt is not absent, examples of just punishment are lacking? We have sinned as much as anyone, but we alone are being punished. Alone, I say; for I dare assert that if the punishments of all the centuries, subsequent to that most famous ark that bore the remains of mortals over unformed seas, were compared to present ones, they would resemble delightful activities, games, and moments of ease. Nor is it fitting to compare these misfortunes to any wars, for in such wars there are many kinds of remedies, and ultimately the possibility of at least dying in a manly fashion. For to die well is an exceptional consolation for death. In the present case there is absolutely no remedy, and no comfort. Not knowing the cause and origin of our misfortune only adds to the extent of the disaster. For neither our ignorance nor indeed the plague itself is more troublesome than the nonsense and stories of certain men who profess to know everything, but really know nothing. Their mouths, accustomed to falsehoods, are finally silenced, and where at first they emitted their ignorance as is their custom, they finally remain closed with stupor. But let me return to my inquiry.

Is it not true that just as for wayfarers one part of the road produces a weariness that is admitted only upon reaching another part, so does it happen to us that Your mercy, oh Lord, gradually exhausted by human faults, and depressed by the continuing increase in such faults, finally can take no more, and must subside, and that You, like an ideal wayfarer unable to endure any more have cast us behind You and angrily turned away the eyes of Your mercy? But if this is so, we suffer punishment not only for our sins but for those of our fathers. I do not know whether we are worse than they, but certainly we are more wretched. Or is it perhaps true as is suspected by certain great minds that God cares not for mortal things? Let such madness not even enter our minds: if You did not care they would not be. What must be our opinion of those who attribute our welfare not to God but to nature, when we have been dedicated to the study of Your truths? Even [Roman writer] Seneca calls most ungrateful those who through a change of name disguise a function of God, and through impious mockery deny what is owed to divine majesty. You certainly do care for us and our affairs, oh God, but the causes are concealed and unknown to us as to why we have been judged by You the most worthy of all centuries to be punished most harshly without there being any lessening of Your justice because it is hidden from us. For the depth of Your judgments is inscrutable and inaccessible to human senses. Therefore either we are really the worst of all, something which I would like to but dare not deny, or else we are being saved through these present evils by becoming more experienced and more pure for future blessings, or else there is something involved which we are simply unable to fathom. Yet, whatever the causes may be, however much you conceal them, the effects are most visible.

Vanishing Comrades

But to turn from public to private grief, the first part of the second year is hardly over since tearfully I left you crying at the mouth of the Sorgue as I returned to Italy. I am not asking you to consider a long period of time; consider simply these very few days and call to mind what we were and what we are. Where are our sweet friends now, where are their beloved faces, where are their soothing words, where is their mild and pleasant conversation? What thunderbolt destroyed all those things, what earthquake overturned them, what storm overcame them, what abyss absorbed them? We used to be a crowd, now we are almost alone. We must seek new friendships. But where or for what reason when the human species is almost extinct and the end, as I hope, is near? Why pretend, dear brother, for we are indeed alone. I believe that it was God's purpose to strip us of the sweet charms and impediments of this life so that we might now more freely desire the next life. See where we have arrived as a result of the sudden changes! We are now in a position to test that saying of [the Greek philosopher] Epicurus: "We represent a sufficiently large theater one for the other." To be truthful to each other, how long will we be able to say this? Or what soothsayer can indicate the extent to which we can have faith in the stability of such a reciprocal theater, when on the other hand we see the columns already shaking? About what can I in writing this be more certain concerning your life than you, in reading this, can be concerning mine? Man is too frail and proud an animal, he builds too securely on fragile foundations. See to what a small number we have been reduced from so large a group of comrades: and note that while we are speaking we ourselves are also fleeing and are vanishing in the fashion of shades, and in a moment of time one of us receives the news of the departure of the other and the survivor will in turn be following upon the footsteps of the other. What are we, therefore, dearest brother? What are we, indeed? Of what do we continue to be proud? Dismayed by his torments, [the Roman orator] Cicero says in one of his letters to Atticus, "What are we or how long shall we be attending to these things?" Indeed a brief but good question, if I am not mistaken. It is also a wholesome question, pregnant with useful advice in which the alert digger will discover a great deal about true humility and modesty and great contempt for fleeting things. I say, what are we? How heavy, how slow, how fragile is our body, how confused and how restless is our mind, how changeable and how uncertain and voluble is our destiny? How long shall we be concerned about these things? Very briefly. Cicero certainly meant nothing more by this than had he said: "How long shall we continue to be the very thing we are?" By heavens, certainly not long, since just as this very being of ours cannot last long, so can it actually cease as we utter these very words. Nor should it prove astonishing if this were to happen. Therefore, oh Marcus Tullius, you ask both questions well and seriously. But I ask you, where have you left the third question which is in fact more dangerous and more worthy of being asked? What shall we be after terminating our life here? An important and doubtful matter, indeed, but certainly neglected! Farewell.

The Papal City Is Stricken by Plague

Anonymous Clergyman

> The great fear of the plague was worsened by the realization that nobody, no matter their wealth or their station in life, was safe. The sickness reached rich and poor alike. Kings and their courts were affected, as were doctors and philosophers as well as the highest religious authorities.
>
> In 1348, the plague arrived in the city of Avignon (in what is now southern France), where the court of the pope, the head of the Christian church, had moved from Rome in 1309. An anonymous cleric of the Low Countries, who was visiting Avignon during the plague outbreak, told of what he saw in the following letter dated April 27, 1348. The writer describes the plague's horrible symptoms, the possible causes of the disease (including the deliberate poisoning of the water wells), the flight of people who believed they were safer in the countryside, and the reactions of the papal authorities including Pope Clement VI.

The disease is threefold in its infection; that is to say, firstly, men suffer in their lungs and breathing, and whoever have these corrupted, or even slightly attacked, cannot by any means escape nor live beyond two days. Examinations have been made by doctors in many cities of Italy, and also in Avignon, by order of the Pope, in order to discover the origin of this disease. Many dead bodies have been thus opened and dissected, and it is found that all who

Francis Aidan Gasquet, *The Black Death of 1348 and 1349*. London: George Bell and Sons, 1908.

have died thus suddenly have had their lungs infected and have spat blood. The contagious nature of the disease is indeed the most terrible of all the terrors (of the time), for when anyone who is infected by it dies, all who see him in his sickness, or visit him, or do any business with him, or even carry him to the grave, quickly follow him thither, and there is no known means of protection.

There is another form of the sickness, however, at present running its course concurrently with the first; that is, certain aposthumes [tumors] appear under both arms, and by these also people quickly die. A third form of the disease—like the two former, running its course at this same time with them—is that from which people of both sexes suffer from aposthumes in the groin. This, likewise, is quickly fatal. The sickness has already grown to such proportions that, from fear of contagion, no doctor will visit a sick man, even if the invalid would gladly give him everything he possessed; neither does a father visit his son, nor a mother her daughter, nor a brother his brother, nor a son his father, nor a friend his friend, nor an acquaintance his acquaintance, nor, in fact, does anyone go to another, no matter how closely he may be allied to him by blood, unless he is prepared to die with him or quickly to follow after him. Still, a large number of persons have died merely through their affection for others; for they might have escaped had they not, moved by piety and Christian charity, visited the sick at the time.

To put the matter shortly, one-half, or more than a half, of the people at Avignon are already dead. Within the walls of the city there are now more than 7,000 houses shut up; in these no one is living, and all who have inhabited them are departed; the suburbs hardly contain any people at all. A field near 'Our Lady of Miracles' has been bought by the Pope and consecrated as a cemetery. In this, from the 13th of March, 11,000 corpses have been buried. This number does not include those interred in the cemetery of the hospital of St. Anthony, in cemeteries belonging to the religious bodies, and in the many others which exist in Avignon. Nor must I be silent about the neighbouring parts, for at Marseilles all the gates of the city, with the exception of two small ones, are now closed, for there four-fifths of the inhabitants are dead.

The like account I can give of all the cities and towns of Provence [a region in southern France]. Already the sickness has crossed the Rhone [River], and ravaged many cities and villages as far as Toulouse, and it ever increases in violence as it proceeds. On account of this great mortality there

The Pope's Physician Observes the Plague

In his book La Grande Chirurgie, *Guy de Chauliac, the official physician to Pope Clement VI at Avignon, noted his observations of the epidemic and revealed that he was one of the rare few who, "by the will of God," lived to tell of coming down with the bubonic plague.*

The great mortality appeared at Avignon in January, 1348, when I was in the service of Pope Clement VI. It was of two kinds. The first lasted two months, with continued fever and spitting of blood, and people died of it in three days. The second was all the rest of the time, also with continuous fever, and with tumors in the external parts, chiefly the armpits and groin; and people died in five days. It was so contagious, especially [when] accompanied by spitting of blood, that not only by staying together, but even by looking at one another, people caught it, with the result that men died without attendants and were buried without priests. The father did not visit his son, nor the son his father. Charity was dead and hope crushed.

I call it great, because it covered the whole world, or lacked little of doing so. For it began in the East, and thus casting its darts against the world, passed through our region toward the West. It was so great that it left scarcely a fourth part of the people. And I say that it was such that its like has never been heard tell of before; of the pestilences in the past that we read of, none was so great as this. For those covered is such a fear of death that people do not dare even to speak with anyone whose relative has died, because it is frequently remarked that in a family where one dies nearly all the relations follow him, and this is commonly believed among the people. Neither are the sick now served by their kindred, except as dogs would be; food is put near the bed for them to eat and drink, and then those still in health fly and leave the house. When a man dies some rough countrymen, called

---

only one region, this the whole world; those could be treated in some way, this in none.

For this reason it was useless and shameful for the doctors, the more so as they dared not visit the sick, for fear of being infected. And when they did visit them, they did hardly anything for them, and were paid nothing; for all the sick died, except some few at the last who escaped, the buboes being ripened.

Many were in doubt about the cause of this great mortality. In some places, they thought that the Jews had poisoned the world: and so they killed them. In others, that it was the poor deformed: and they drove them out. In others, that it was the nobles: and they feared to go abroad. Finally they reached the point where they kept guards in the cities and villages, and permitted the entry of no one who was not well known. And if powders or unguents were found on anyone the owners, for fear that they were poisons, were forced to swallow them. . . .

And I, to avoid infamy, dared not absent myself, but with continual fear preserved myself as best I could by means of the [available] remedies. Notwithstanding this, toward the end of the mortality I fell into a continuous fever, with a tumor in the groin. I was ill for nearly six weeks, and was in such great danger that all my associates thought that I would die; but the tumor being ripened, and treated as I have said, I escaped by the will of God.

Anna Montgomery Campbell, *The Black Death and Men of Learning.* New York: Columbia University Press, 1931.

gavoti, come to the house, and, after receiving a sufficiently large reward, carry the corpse to the grave. Neither relatives nor friends go to the sick, nor do priests even hear their confessions nor give them the Sacraments; but everyone whilst still in health looks after himself. It daily happens that some rich man dying is borne to the grave by these ruffians without lights, and without a soul to follow him, except these hired mourners. When a corpse is carried by all fly through the streets and get into their houses. Nor do these said wretched *gavoti*, strong as they are, escape; but most of them after a time become infected by this contagion and die. All the poor who were wont to receive bread from the rich are dead; that is to say, briefly, where daily in ordinary times there were distributed sixty-four measures of wheat for bread, fifty loaves being made from each measure, now only one measure is given away, and sometimes even a half is found to be sufficient.

The Pope Gives Absolution

And it is said that altogether in three months—that is from January 25th to the present day (April 27th)—62,000 bodies have been buried in Avignon. The Pope, however, about the middle of March last past, after mature deliberation, gave plenary absolution till Easter, as far as the keys of the Church extended, to all those who, having confessed and being contrite, should happen to die of the sickness. He ordered likewise devout processions, singing the Litanies, to be made on certain days each week, and to these, it is said, people sometimes come from the neighbouring districts to the number of 2,000; amongst them many of both sexes are barefooted, some are in sackcloth, some with ashes, walking with tears, and tearing their hair, and beating themselves with scourges even to the drawing of blood. The Pope was personally present at some of these processions, but they were then within the precincts of his palace. What will be the end, or whence all this has had its beginning, God alone knows. . . .

Some wretched men have been caught with certain dust, and, whether justly or unjustly God only knows, they are accused of having poisoned the water, and men in fear do not drink the water from wells; for this many have been burnt and daily are burnt.

Fish, even sea fish, is commonly not eaten, as people say they have been infected by the bad air. Moreover, people do not eat, nor even touch spices, which have not been kept a year, since they fear they may have lately arrived in the aforesaid ships. And, indeed, it has many times been observed that those who have eaten these new spices and even some kinds of sea fish have suddenly been taken ill.

I write this to you, my friends, that you may know the dangers in which we live. And if you desire to preserve yourselves, the best advice is to eat and drink temperately, to avoid cold, not to commit excess of any kind, and, above all, to converse little with others, at this time especially, except with the few whose breath is sweet. But it is best to remain at home until this epidemic has passed. . . .

Know, also, that the Pope has lately left Avignon, as is reported, and has gone to the castle called Stella, near Valence on the Rhone, two leagues off, to remain there till times change. The Curia, however, preferred to remain at Avignon, (but) vacations have been proclaimed till the feast of St. Michael. All the auditors, advocates, and procurators have either left, intend to leave immediately, or are dead. I am in the hands of God, to whom I commend myself. My master will follow the Pope, so they say, and I with him, for there are some castles near the airy mountains where the mortality has not appeared, and it is thought that the best chance is there. To choose and to do what is best may the Omnipotent and merciful God grant us all. Amen.

The Plague Ravages France

Jean de Venette

For the chroniclers of the fourteenth century, the plague represented one of the worst occurrences of a morbid and calamitous era. After famines and disease outbreaks in the early decades of the century, a disastrous war had begun between the English and French. While a poor climate had affected crops and harvests, thousands of people died of starvation in France, one of the wealthiest realms of Europe.

Jean de Venette, a friar of the Carmelite order and a master of theology at the University of Paris, wrote a long account of these miseries in the late fourteenth century. In contrast to many of his contemporaries, Venette gives a balanced and unbiased report of the plague, of the beliefs of the people on the origins of the plague, the effects of the plague on common people as well as kings and nobles, and the rise of the sect of flagellants in the year 1349.

In A.D. 1348, the people of France and of almost the whole world were struck by a blow other than war. For in addition to the famine which I described in the beginning and to the wars which I described in the course of this narrative, pestilence and its attendant tribulations appeared again in various parts of the world. In the month of August, 1348, after Vespers when the sun was beginning to set, a big and very bright star appeared above Paris, toward the west. It did not seem, as stars usually do, to be very high above our

Jean de Venette, *The Chronicle of Jean de Venette*, translated by Jean Birdsall and edited by Richard A. Newhall. Now York: Columbia University Press, 1953. Copyright © 1953 by Columbia University Press. Reproduced by permission.

hemisphere but rather very near. As the sun set and night came on, this star did not seem to me or to many other friars who were watching it to move from one place. At length, when night had come, this big star, to the amazement of all of us who were watching, broke into many different rays and, as it shed these rays over Paris toward the east, totally disappeared and was completely annihilated. Whether it was a comet or not, whether it was composed of airy exhalations and was finally resolved into vapor, I leave to the decision of astronomers. It is, however, possible that it was a presage of the amazing pestilence to come, which, in fact, followed very shortly in Paris and throughout France and elsewhere, as I shall tell. All this year and the next, the mortality of men and women, of the young even more than of the old, in Paris and in the kingdom of France, and also, it is said, in other parts of the world, was so great that it was almost impossible to bury the dead. People lay ill little more than two or three days and died suddenly, as it were in full health. He who was well one day was dead the next and being carried to his grave. Swellings appeared suddenly in the armpit or in the groin—in many cases both—and they were infallible signs of death. This sickness or pestilence was called an epidemic by the doctors. Nothing like the great numbers who died in the years 1348 and 1349 has been heard of or seen or read of in times past. This plague and disease came from *ymaginatione* or association and contagion, for if a well man visited the sick he only rarely evaded the risk of death. Wherefore in many towns timid priests withdrew, leaving the exercise of their ministry to such of the religious as were more daring. In many places not two out of twenty remained alive. So high was the mortality at the Hôtel-Dieu [a hospital] in Paris that for a long time, more than five hundred dead were carried daily with great devotion in carts to the cemetery of the Holy Innocents in Paris for burial. A very great number of the saintly sisters of the Hôtel-Dieu who, not fearing to die, nursed the sick in all sweetness and humility, with no thought of honor, a number too often renewed by death, rest in peace with Christ, as we may piously believe.

This plague, it is said, began among the unbelievers, came to Italy, and then crossing the Alps reached Avignon, where it attacked several cardinals and took from them their whole household. Then it spread, unforeseen, to France, through Gascony and Spain, little by little, from town to town, from village to village, from house to house, and finally from person to person. It even crossed over to Germany, though it was not so bad there as with us. During the epidemic, God of His accustomed goodness deigned to grant this grace, that however suddenly men died, almost all awaited death joyfully. Nor was there anyone who died without confessing his sins and receiving the holy viaticum [last rites]. To the even greater benefit of the dying, Pope Clement VI through their confessors mercifully gave and granted absolution from penalty to the dying in many cities and fortified towns. Men died the more willingly for this and left many inheritances and temporal goods to churches and monastic orders, for in many cases they had seen their close heirs and children die before them.

Poisoning the Wells

Some said that this pestilence was caused by infection of the air and waters, since there was at this time no famine nor lack of food supplies, but on the contrary great abundance. As a result of this theory of infected water and air as the source of the plague the Jews were suddenly and violently charged with infecting wells and water and corrupting the air. The whole world rose up against them cruelly on this account. In Germany and other parts of the world where Jews lived, they were massacred and slaughtered by Christians, and many thousands were burned everywhere, indiscriminately. The unshaken, if fatuous, constancy of the men and their wives was remarkable. For mothers hurled their children first into the fire that they might not be baptized and then leaped in after them to burn with their husbands and children. It is said that many bad Christians were found who in a like manner put poison into wells. But in truth, such poisonings, granted that they actually were perpetrated, could not have caused so great a plague nor have infected so many people. There were other causes; for example, the will of God and the corrupt humors and evil inherent in air and earth. Perhaps the poisonings, if they actually took place in some localities, reenforced these causes. The plague lasted in France for the greater part of the years 1348 and 1349 and then ceased. Many country villages and many houses in good towns remained empty and deserted. Many houses, including some splendid dwellings, very soon fell into ruins. Even in Paris several houses were thus ruined, though fewer here than elsewhere.

After the cessation of the epidemic, pestilence, or plague, the men and women who survived married each other. There was no sterility among the women, but on the contrary fertility beyond the ordinary. Pregnant women were seen on every side. Many twins were born and even three children at once. But the most surprising fact is that children born after the plague, when they became of an age for teeth, had only twenty or twenty-two teeth, though before that time men commonly had thirty-two in their upper and lower jaws together. What this diminution in the number of teeth signified I wonder greatly, unless it be a new era resulting from the destruction of one human generation by the plague and its replacement by another. But woe is me! the world was not changed for the better but for the worse by this renewal of population. For men were more avaricious and grasping than before, even though they had far greater possessions. They were more covetous and disturbed each other more frequently with suits, brawls, disputes, and pleas. Nor by the mortality resulting from this terrible plague inflicted by God was peace between kings and lords established. On the contrary, the enemies of the king of France and of the Church were stronger and wickeder than before and stirred up wars on sea and on land. Greater evils than before pullulated everywhere in the world. And this fact was very remarkable. Although there was an abundance of all goods, yet everything was twice as dear, whether it were utensils, victuals, or merchandise, hired helpers or peasants and serfs, except for some hereditary domains which remained abundantly stocked with everything. Charity began to cool, and iniquity with ignorance and sin to abound, for few could be found in the good towns and castles who knew how or were willing to instruct children in the rudiments of grammar. . . .

The Flagellant Sect Arises

In the year 1349, while the plague was still active and spreading from town to town, men in Germany, Flanders, Hainaut, and Lorraine uprose and began a new sect on their own authority. Stripped to the waist, they gathered in large groups and bands and marched in procession through the crossroads and squares of cities and good towns. There they formed circles and beat upon their backs with weighted scourges, rejoicing as they did so in loud voices and singing hymns suitable to their rite and newly composed for it. Thus for thirty-three days they marched through many towns doing their penance and affording a great spectacle to the wondering people. They flogged their shoulders and arms with scourges tipped with iron points so zealously as to draw blood. But they did not come to Paris nor to any part of France, for they were forbidden to do so by the king of France, who did not want them. He acted on the advice of the masters of theology of the University of Paris, who said that this new sect had been formed contrary to the will of God, to the rites of Holy Mother Church, and to the salvation of all their souls. That indeed this was and is true appeared shortly. For Pope Clement VI was fully informed concerning this fatuous new rite by the masters of Paris through emissaries reverently sent to him and, on the grounds that it had been damnably formed, contrary to law, he forbade the Flagellants under threat of anathema to practise in the future the public penance which they had so presumptuously undertaken. His prohibition was just, for the Flagellants, supported by certain fatuous priests and monks, were enunciating doctrines and opinions which were beyond measure evil, erroneous, and fallacious. For example, they said that their blood thus drawn by the scourge and poured out was mingled with the blood of Christ. Their many errors showed how little they knew of the Catholic faith. Wherefore, as they had begun fatuously of themselves and not of God, so in a short time they were reduced to nothing. On being warned, they desisted and humbly received absolution and penance at the hands of their prelates as the pope's representatives. Many honorable women and devout matrons, it must be added, had done this penance with scourges, marching and singing through towns and churches like the men, but after a little like the others they desisted.

Chapter 3

Explaining and Contending with the Plague

Chapter Preface

The victims of the Black Death sought an explanation for the terrible disease visited upon them. They had reason to hope that the explanation could be found. In recent times, scientific inquiry had flourished. The first universities of Europe were founded during the twelfth century. Lecturers at these universities questioned many of the doctrines of the church, which remained the dominant institution in society. Christianity was their faith—but their quest was to learn how the Christian God had created and ordered the natural world.

While ordinary people looked to the Bible and their faith for the answer to the unstoppable pestilence, doctors and scientists could not agree on the true cause. Some explained it as an astronomical event, noting that the planets had recently entered an unlucky alignment in the heavens. Others blamed miasmic vapors belched up from underneath the surface of the earth by earthquakes, volcanic explosions, and other catastrophic events.

Doctors debated over the best means of preventing the plague. Some argued for a strict diet of one sort or another, and others advised a change in lifestyle. For those who fell victim of the plague, doctors offered a wide variety of prescriptions and preparations. None seemed to work.

The microscope was not yet invented, and what could be seen with the naked eye was all that could truly be seen. For this reason, bacteria and viruses were still unknown, and the bacillus that causes the plague remained invisible. For all their learning, reason, and intelligence, the thinkers of the fourteenth century were still hampered by medieval technology, which was not yet capable of revealing the true nature of contagious diseases.

Worldly Evils Brought the Plague

Heinrich von Herford

> Bewildered by the death and the fear surrounding them, the people of Europe searched for a cause for the Black Death. The members of the clergy, predisposed to seeing in all natural events the hand of God, understood the plague as a divine retribution. For churchmen and lay people alike, the Black Death could mean only one thing: God's punishment for mortal sin, believed by many in the fourteenth century to have reached a feverish pitch.
>
> Like many others, Heinrich von Herford, a German monk of the Dominican order, believed the root cause of the plague to be the corruption and evil practices of the clergy. Herford was not alone, for example, in condemning the sale of clerical offices and privileges, a common practice throughout Europe. But in the chronicle that follows, written some years after the Black Death, he also recounts the sins of secular rulers and lords who fought over money, property, and titles. Herford describes the many natural disasters that followed from this corruption—not only plague but also earthquakes and a rain of toads and snakes.

A t this time violent disagreements, rebellions, conspiracies, plots and intrigues sprang up among both secular and regular clergy everywhere, just as the apostle retold in 2 Timothy 3 and 2 Corinthians 12. At the same time there were also other disturbances, of young against old, ignoble against noble, and an unusual degree of unrest (whether general or specific) in many cities, monasteries and congregations. The heresy of simony [the sale of clerical offices by the church] also grew so strong among the clergy, and overwhelmed them so completely, that everyone, of whatever degree (great, middling or humble) and of whatever status (secular or regular) in some fashion openly bought and sold spiritualities of all sorts. They did not blush for shame, they were not reproved or criticised by anyone, let alone punished, so that it might seem as if the Lord, far from expelling the buyers and sellers from the temple, had made them at home there, or as if simony was now to be judged not heretical but ecclesiastical, catholic and holy. They traded prebends, benefices [income-producing property granted to the church by a government or feudal landowner], and all other ecclesiastical dignities, parish churches; chapels, vicarages and altars for money, women and sometimes for concubines; they staked them, lost and won them, on a game of dice.

Then there were many disturbances over contested kingdoms, principalities, archbishoprics, bishoprics, prebends and other things of that kind, such as between the Emperor Lewis, Charles King of Bohemia and Count Gunther of Schwarzburg over who was to be King of the Romans [Holy Roman Emperor]; between John, King of France and Edward, King of England over the kingdom of France; and between rival claimants for the archbishopric of Mainz and for Bremen, Minden, Hildesheim, Halberstadt, Worms, Schleswig and many others. Prebends, dignities and inordinate numbers of lesser posts were neglected.

Then each religious order was wrenched asunder by its members, as the birth of vipers tears apart the maternal womb. Every office and appointment among them could only be secured by money, or favouritism, or some other useful gift. Just as once prebends and dignities of that sort were sought and obtained from prelates or in the Roman Curia, so the offices of abbot, prior, warden, master, lector, definitor, and everything else, however petty, was bought, occupied and held by whoever possessed the necessary money (by theft or some other means), regardless of whether they were foul tempered, boorish, illiterate, under age, inexperienced, stupid, or lacking in any other way whatsoever. And in these days distinguished people cannot easily be found (as was once the case) among the secular and regular clergy. Look at all these abbots, priors, wardens, masters, lectors, provosts and canons, and groan! Look at their life, the example they give, their career and their doctrine, and at the risks to their people, and tremble! And you too, Lord, father of mercies, look down and have mercy, for we have sinned against you.

In the 31st year of Emperor Lewis, around the feast of the Conversion of St Paul [25 January] there was an earthquake throughout Carinthia and Carniola [regions of present-day Austria] which was so severe that everyone feared for their lives. There were repeated shocks, and on one night the earth shook 20 times. Sixteen cities were destroyed and their inhabitants killed. One city, called Cencenighe, was entirely destroyed along with the Franciscan friary there and not one man escaped. And in many places it is hard to believe that anyone ever lived there. Thirty-six mountain fortresses and their inhabitants were destroyed and it has been calculated that more than 40,000 men were swallowed up or overwhelmed. Two very high mountains, with a highway between them, were hurled together, so that there can never be a road there again. This information comes from a letter of the house of Friesach to the provincial prior of Germany. It says in the same letter that in this year fire falling from heaven consumed the land of the Turks for 16 days; that for a few days it rained toads and snakes, by which many men were killed; that a pestilence has gathered strength in many parts of the world; that not one man in ten escaped in Marseilles; that all the Franciscans there have died; that beyond Rome the city of Messina [in Sicily, where the plague arrived in Europe] has been largely deserted because of the pestilence. And a knight coming from that place said that he did not find five men alive there. All these things from the same letter.

Planetary Conjunctions and the Corruption of Air

Medical Faculty of the University of Paris

> While the plague raged through their cities, the rulers of
> Europe called on the leading men of science and medicine to
> provide an explanation and suggestions on how to fight the
> disease. In France, King Philip VI turned to the most respected
> institution of learning in Europe, the University of Paris. King
> Philip called on the university's faculty of medicine to consult
> together and then give a detailed report of their findings.
>
> The Paris faculty responded in June 1348 with the following
> tract, explaining how the conjunction of stars and planets in the
> heavens, and the corruption of the air on Earth, had caused the
> Black Death. The faculty also pointed out that the recent unac-
> customed nature of the seasons, which had not run their usual
> course, provided clear signs of the pestilence to come. Along
> with suggestions for how to avoid and treat the disease, the fac-
> ulty recommends that the people of the kingdom who search
> for a cure return humbly to God for human salvation.

Seeing things which cannot be explained, even by the
most gifted intellects, initially stirs the human mind to
amazement; but after marvelling, the prudent soul next
yields to its desire for understanding and, anxious for its
own perfection, strives with all its might to discover the
causes of the amazing events. For there is within the human

Medical Faculty of the University of Paris, "Report of the Paris Medical Faculty, October
1348," translated and edited by Rosemary Horrox, *The Black Death*. Manchester, UK:
Manchester University Press, 1994. Copyright © 1994 by Rosemary Horrox. Reproduced
by permission of the publisher.

mind an innate desire to seize on goodness and truth. As the Philosopher [i.e., Aristotle] makes plain, all things seek for the good and want to understand. To attain this end we have listened to the opinions of many modern experts on astrology and medicine about the causes of the epidemic which has prevailed since 1345. However, because their conclusions still leave room for considerable uncertainty, we, the masters of the faculty of medicine at Paris, inspired by the command of the most illustrious prince, our most serene lord, Philip, King of France, and by our desire to achieve something of public benefit, have decided to compile, with God's help, a brief compendium of the distant and immediate causes of the present universal epidemic (as far as these can be understood by the human intellect) and of wholesome remedies; drawing on the opinions of the most brilliant ancient philosophers and modern experts, astronomers as well as doctors of medicine. . . .

Concerning the Universal and Distant Cause

We say that the distant and first cause of this pestilence was and is the configuration of the heavens. In 1345, at one hour after noon on 20 March, there was a major conjunction of three planets in Aquarius. This conjunction, along with other earlier conjunctions and eclipses, by causing a deadly corruption of the air around us, signifies mortality and famine—and also other things about which we will not speak here because they are not relevant. Aristotle testifies that this is the case in his book *Concerning the causes of the properties of the elements*, in which he says that mortality of races and the depopulation of kingdoms occur at the conjunction of Saturn and Jupiter, for great events then arise, their nature depending on the trigon in which the conjunction occurs. And this is found in ancient philosophers, and Albertus Magnus [a thirteenth-century philosopher who was considered the greatest scientist of his day] in his book, *Concerning the causes of the properties of the elements* (treatise 2, chapter 1) says that the conjunction of Mars and

Jupiter causes a great pestilence in the air, especially when they come together in a hot, wet sign [such as Aquarius], as was the case in 1345. For Jupiter, being wet and hot, draws up evil vapours from the earth and Mars, because it is immoderately hot and dry, then ignites the vapours, and as a result there were lightnings, sparks, noxious vapours and fires throughout the air.

These effects were intensified because Mars—a malevolent planet, breeding anger and wars—was in the sign of Leo from 6 October 1347 until the end of May this year, along with the head of the dragon, and because all these things are hot they attracted many vapours; which is why the winter was not as cold as it should have been. And Mars was also retrograde and therefore attracted many vapours from the earth and the sea which, when mixed with the air, corrupted its substance. Mars was also looking upon Jupiter with a hostile aspect, that is to say quartile, and that caused an evil disposition or quality in the air, harmful and hateful to our nature. This state of affairs generated strong winds (for according to Albertus in the first book of his *Meteora*, Jupiter has the property of raising powerful winds, particularly from the south) which gave rise to excess heat and moisture on the earth; although in fact it was the dampness which was most marked in our part of the world. And this is enough about the distant or universal cause for the moment.

The Particular and Near Cause

Although major pestilential illnesses can be caused by the corruption of water or food, as happens at times of famine and infertility, yet we still regard illnesses proceeding from the corruption of the air as much more dangerous. This is because bad air is more noxious than food or drink in that it can penetrate quickly to the heart and lungs to do its damage. We believe that the present epidemic or plague has arisen from air corrupt in its substance, and not changed in its attributes. By which we wish it be understood that air, being pure and clear by nature, can only become putrid or corrupt by being mixed with something else, that is to say, with evil vapours.

What happened was that the many vapours which had been corrupted at the time of the conjunction were drawn up from the earth and water, and were then mixed with the air and spread abroad by frequent gusts of wind in the wild southerly gales, and because of these alien vapours which they carried the winds corrupted the air in its substance, and are still doing so. And this corrupted air, when breathed in, necessarily penetrates to the heart and corrupts the substance of the spirit there and rots the surrounding moisture, and the heat thus caused destroys the life force, and this is the immediate cause of the present epidemic.

And moreover these winds, which have become so common here, have carried among us (and may perhaps continue to do so in future) bad, rotten and poisonous vapours from elsewhere: from swamps, lakes and chasms, for instance, and also (which is even more dangerous) from unburied or unburnt corpses—which might well have been a cause of the epidemic. Another possible cause of corruption, which needs to be borne in mind, is the escape of the rottenness trapped in the centre of the earth as a result of earthquakes—something which has indeed recently occurred. But the conjunctions could have been the universal and distant cause of all these harmful things, by which air and water have been corrupted.

Concerning Prognostication and Signs

Unseasonable weather is a particular cause of illness. For the ancients, notably Hippocrates, are agreed that if the four seasons run awry, and do not keep their proper course, then plagues and mortal passions are engendered that year. Experience tells us that for some time the seasons have not succeeded each other in the proper way. Last winter was not as cold as it should have been, with a great deal of rain; the spring windy and latterly wet. Summer was late, not as hot as it should have been, and extremely wet—the weather very changeable from day to day, and hour to hour; the air often troubled, and then still again, looking as if it was going to rain but then not doing so. Autumn too was very rainy and misty. It is because the whole year here—or most of it—was warm and wet that the air is pestilential. For it is a sign of pestilence for the air to be warm and wet at unseasonable times. Wherefore we may fear a future pestilence here, which is particularly from the root beneath [i.e., from earthly causes], because it is subject to the evil impress of the heavens, especially since that conjunction was in a western sign. Therefore if next winter is very rainy and less cold than it ought to be, we should expect an epidemic round about late winter and spring—and if it occurs it will be long and dangerous, for usually unseasonable weather is of only brief duration, but when it lasts over many seasons, as has obviously been the case here, it stands to reason that its effects will be longer-lasting and more dangerous, unless ensuing seasons change their nature in the opposite way. Thus if the winter in the north turns out to be cold and dry, the plagues might be arrested.

We have not said that the future pestilence will be exceptionally dangerous, for we do not wish to give the impression that it will be as dangerous here as in southern or eastern regions. For the conjunctions and the other causes discussed above had a more immediate impact on those regions than on ours. However, in the judgement of astrologers (who follow [the ancient Greek astronomer] Ptolemy on this) plagues are likely, although not inevitable, because so many exhalations and inflammations have been observed, such as a comet and shooting stars. Also the sky has looked yellow and the air reddish because of the burnt vapours. There has also been much lightning and flashes and frequent thunder, and winds of such violence and strength that they have carried dust storms from the south. These things, and in particular the powerful earthquakes, have done universal harm and left a trail of corruption. There have been masses of dead fish, animals and other things along the sea shore, and in many places trees covered in dust, and some people claim to have seen a multitude of frogs and reptiles generated from the corrupt matter; and all these things seem to have come from the great corruption of the air and earth. All these things have been noted before as signs of plague by numerous wise men who are still remembered with respect and who experienced them themselves.

No wonder, therefore, that we fear that we are in for an epidemic. But it should be noted that in saying this we do not intend to exclude the possibility of illnesses arising from the character of the present year—for as the aphorism of Hippocrates has it: a year of many fogs and damps is a year of many illnesses. On the other hand, the susceptibility of the body of the patient is the most immediate cause in the breeding of illnesses, and therefore no cause is likely to have an effect unless the patient is susceptible to its effects. We must therefore emphasise that although, because everyone has to breathe, everyone will be at risk from the corrupted air, not everyone will be made ill by it but only those, who will no doubt be numerous, who have a susceptibility to it; and very few indeed of those who do succumb will escape.

The bodies most likely to take the stamp of this pestilence are those which are hot and moist, for they are the most susceptible to putrefaction. The following are also more at risk: bodies bunged up with evil humours, because the unconsumed waste matter is not being expelled as it should; those following a bad life style, with too much exercise, sex and bathing; the thin and weak, and persistent worriers; babies, women and young people; and corpulent people with a ruddy complexion. However those with dry bodies, purged of waste matter, who adopt a sensible and suitable regimen, will succumb to the pestilence more slowly.

We must not overlook the fact that any pestilence proceeds from the divine will, and our advice can therefore only be to return humbly to God. But this does not mean forsaking doctors. For the Most High created earthly medicine, and although God alone cures the sick, he does so through the medicine which in his generosity he provided. Blessed be the glorious and high God, who does not refuse his help, but has clearly set out a way of being cured for those who fear him. And this is enough of the third chapter, and of the whole first part.

The Plague Is Caused by Malevolent Spirits

Montpelier Physician

Medieval scientists came up with many theories to explain the origins of plague. Many relied on the theory of corrupted elements—earth, air, fire, and water; others saw the Black Death as an extreme example of the humors of the body—blood, phlegm, yellow bile, and black bile—being out of their normal equilibrium. In the following excerpt, written in 1349, an anonymous physician of the city of Montpelier, France, gives his opinion on the origins of the plague as an evil spirit that travels from the eyes of a sick person to a healthy victim.

This epidemic, according to some people, has the power to kill large numbers by air alone, simply by the breath or the conversation of the sick. They say that the air breathed out by the sick and inhaled by the healthy people round about wounds and kills them, and that this occurs particularly when the sick are on the point of death. But that would kill gradually, after an interval rather than straight away; and the greater strength of this epidemic is such that it kills almost instantly, as soon as the airy spirit leaving the eyes of the sick man has struck the eye of a healthy bystander looking at him, for then the poisonous nature passes from one eye to the other. And this occurs particularly when the sick are at the point of death.

No one who has seen the theories of Euclid concerning burning glasses, and concave and reflecting glasses, will be

Montpelier Physician, "Transmission of the Plague," translated and edited by Rosemary Horrox, *The Black Death*. Manchester, UK: Manchester University Press, 1994. Copyright © 1994 by Rosemary Horrox. Reproduced by permission of the publisher.

surprised by this, but will appreciate that the origins of this epidemic and its ability to pass from the sick to the healthy and to kill them, are natural and not miraculous; for something is only 'miraculous' when it does not have a natural reason or cause. The airy and subtle nature which issues from the heat and brightness of the sun is immediately kindled and flares up when reflected by two mirrors. This is achieved by condensing thin air just using the brightness generated by the sun's rays and the mirrors. That brightness can be used to burn and destroy nearby buildings, houses, castles and trees, and an example of this can be found in Euclid's book. In the same way the corruption of the air has an impact on human bodies, and it has a more immediate impact on them than on other things because of the soft primary matter of which they are compounded. . . .

The Effects of Food and Moisture

[Under-ripe] food inevitably brings sickness, because it ferments in the stomach to create a dangerous viscid and windy moisture, and draws the blood into the liver, which inevitably causes sickness and poisoning. This corrupt matter often forms a windy ulcer, and this is why many such ulcers form on the right side of the body rather than the left. . . .

When the windy moisture has filled one place, it ascends via the jugular vein to the brain, and when it reaches the lungs it fills the pulmonary canals, stopping the movement of the lungs so that they cannot ventilate the heart to cool it. And then the heart grows hot, causing a pestilential fever, and that fever stirs up the humours, which erupt into internal and external ulcers, some of which are caused by the humours and others by wind. Then the brain, in sympathy with the heart because of its motion and sponginess, draws the windy and poisonous moisture from the lungs to itself and then ejects it through the ears. The sufferer experiences a terrific din, like a door being smashed down, which is caused by the primary windiness failing to escape, and then the victims die soon afterwards. But sometimes the brain expels the windy and poisonous matter via the optic nerves at the eyes.

This is agony, and the sick man stares fixedly ahead, as if he cannot move his eyes. Amazingly, as it stands in the eyes, the primary windiness assumes the characteristics of a poisonous vapour, and seeks a new home in some other body, which it

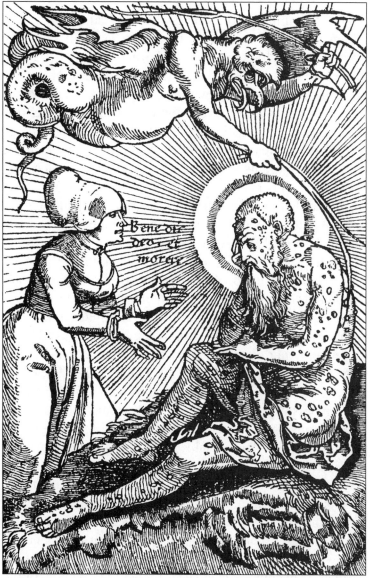

Medieval scientists came up with many theories to explain the plague. This illustration depicts the Black Death as a demon.

can enter and be at rest. And if a healthy person sees this visible vapour, he is stamped with the pestilential illness. The man is poisoned faster than air can leave the sick man, for the thin poison moves faster than the heavy air.

The Basilisk and the Plague

Take the example of the basilisk [a mythical lizard-beast]. Whenever one of these creatures chances upon a healthy person who is looking at it, a visible poisonous vapour passes from the eyes of the basilisk into the eye of the observer, and immediately, without warning, poisons him, or works upon him in some other way so that he is sure to die. And it is a characteristic of the basilisk that it always looks upon the brightest member, that is, the eye. Accordingly, someone who wants to capture a basilisk lights a lantern and sets it above his head, and holds something in front of his eyes, and then the basilisk will choose to look at the light and not at the eyes of his captor, and so can be grabbed and killed. This is also why the weasel, arming itself with rue leaves to protect its eyes, can boldly attack the serpent and kill it. Similarly, the book which Aristotle wrote for Alexander includes the story of a serving girl who was fed on poison by a queen who then sent her to Alexander to kill him by her look and embrace alone. When Aristotle saw the girl he knew by her eyes that she was poisonous and warned Alexander to stay away from her, which he did. They then made a stranger sleep with her, and he died immediately.

From this we may conclude that we should above all take precautions against the gaze and breath of people in the throes of illness. This explains why those in the company of the sick, or employed about them, die so quickly. . . . Therefore when a doctor, priest or friend wants to visit an invalid he should persuade him to close his eyes and then blindfold him with a linen cloth. When this has been done the visitor can treat him, listen to him and handle him in confidence, if he also holds a sponge soaked in vinegar to his nose in hot weather or, in cold weather, keeps his nose in a handful of rue and cummin. And let him also avoid the breath of the invalid.

An Appeal to the Saints and Relics

Michele di Piazza

The first appearance of the plague in 1347 caused fear and panic among the common people of Messina, Sicily. Medical doctors and philosophers could offer little help, and so the people turned to God, to their patron saints, to fervent prayers, and to the healing powers of holy relics to save them from the disease. In this account by Michele di Piazza, the people of Messina appeal to the patriarch of a neighboring town, Catania, for the use of the relics of Saint Agatha. This saint had long been a bone of contention between the two towns, and the disease touched off a bitter feud between people who had already been touched by the plague and those desperate to prevent it.

The account of Michele di Piazza reveals how the Black Death spread from place to place through Sicily, how it completely disrupted daily life, and how the piety of common people seemed to do little to stop it. For the next two years, the experience of the Messinese and the rest of Sicily would be repeated throughout Europe.

In October 1347, at about the beginning of the month, twelve Genoese galleys, fleeing from the divine vengeance which Our Lord had sent upon them for their sins, put into the port of Messina. The Genoese carried such a disease in their bodies that if anyone so much as spoke with one of them he was infected with the deadly illness and could not avoid death. The signs of death among the Genoese, and among the Messinese when they came to share the illness with them, were as follows. Breath spread the infection among those speaking together, with one infecting the other, and it seemed as if the victim was struck all at once by the affliction and was, so to speak, shattered by it. This shattering impact, together with the inhaled infection, caused the eruption of a sort of boil, the size of a lentil, on the thigh or arm, which so infected and invaded the body that the victims violently coughed up blood, and after three days' incessant vomiting, for which there was no remedy, they died—and with them died not only anyone who had talked with them, but also anyone who had acquired or touched or laid hands on their belongings.

The people of Messina, realising that the death racing through them was linked with the arrival of the Genoese galleys, expelled the Genoese from the city and harbour with all speed. But the illness remained in the city and subsequently caused enormous mortality. It bred such loathing that if a son fell ill of the disease his father flatly refused to stay with him, or, if he did dare to come near him, was infected in turn and was sure to die himself after three days. Not just one person in a house died, but the whole household, down to the cats and the livestock, followed their master to death. Because of the scale of the mortality, many Messinese looked to make confession of their sins and to make their wills, but priests, judges and notaries refused to visit them, and if anyone did visit their houses, whether to hear confession or draw up a will, they were soon sure to die themselves. Indeed the [monastic orders of] Franciscans and Dominicans, and others who were willing to visit the sick to hear their confession and impose penance, died in such large numbers that their priories were all but deserted. What more is there to say? Corpses lay unattended in their own homes. No priests, sons, fathers or kinsmen dared to enter; instead they paid porters large sums to carry the bodies to burial. The houses of the dead stood open, with all the jewels, money and treasure in full view, and if someone wanted to enter there was nothing to stop them; for the plague struck so suddenly that at first there weren't enough officials and then there were none at all.

Catania Defends Its Holy Relics

The Messinese, observing this terrible and unnatural event, chose to leave the city rather than stay and die. Not only did they refuse to enter the city; they did not want to be anywhere near it, but camped with their families in the open air among the vineyards outside the city. Some, indeed the majority, went to the city of Catania, believing that the blessed virgin Agatha of Catania would save them from the disease. From Catania Queen Elisabetta of Sicily ordered her son Federico, who was then in Messina, to join her quickly and he arrived promptly with Venetian galleys.

Several of the Messinese in Catania addressed pious requests to the Patriarch, all begging that he would personally carry the relics of the virgin Agatha to Messina with all due honour. 'For we believe', they said, 'that if the relics come to Messina the city will be saved completely from this disease.' The Patriarch, deeply moved by their prayers, agreed that he would come in person to Messina with the relics. This was about the end of November, 1347. The holy virgin Agatha, aware of the deep seated deceit and cunning of the Messinese (who have always wanted to keep the virgin's relics at Messina and were capable of exploiting the calamity to that end), directed her prayers to God, who arranged it that the whole body of citizens took themselves off to the Patriarch, clamouring and shouting that they did not like this plan at all; and, wresting the keys from the keeper of the church, they roundly abused the Patriarch, declaring that they would see him dead before they let the relics go to Messina.

Confronted by this uproar the Patriarch could not carry out his plan, and accordingly he entered the place where the relics were kept, with all possible devotion and honour, and to the accompaniment of religious chants and prayers he laved some of the holy relics with pure water, and announced that he would take the holy water with him when he travelled to Messina. . . .

Driving Out the Demons

What more is there to say? The Patriarch duly arrived in Messina with the holy water and cured all sorts of sick people in great numbers by sprinkling them with the water and making the sign of the cross. The citizens of Messina flocked to see him, hastening to him with great rejoicing and offering many thanks to him and to God. For demons were manifesting themselves in the city in the likeness of dogs, which inflicted great harm on the bodies of the Messinese. Numb with terror, no man dared leave home. However, at the bidding of the Archbishop of Messina, and with general approval, they all agreed to process around the city with devout litanies. Just

The Plague and the Church

Author Norman Cantor, one of the leading modern historians of the medieval period, confronts the Black Death in his recent book In the Wake of the Plague. *In the following passage, Cantor details some of the effects of the epidemic on the Christian church and the religious practices of the survivors.*

The biomedical devastation had a strange and complex impact on the Church. It may have reinforced a trend away from optimism to pessimism, from a God who could be partly encapsulated in reason and was a mighty comfort and fortress, to one whose majesty and planning and rationale were impenetrable, although that pessimistic inclination was already rising in intellectual circles thirty years before the Great Pestilence.

The century after the Black Death was marked—in England, France, the Low Countries, and Germany—by what may be called the privatization of medieval Christianity. This took both organizational and spiritual forms. Organizationally there was a rush by the affluent upper middle class to as all the people were entering the city a black dog appeared in their midst, carrying a naked sword in its paw. It rushed raging into the church, and broke and smashed all the silver vessels, lamps and candlesticks on the altars. At this sight everyone, half dead with terror, prostrated themselves. When, after some hesitation, they got up again they saw the dog leaving the church, but no one dared to follow it or go near it.

The Messinese, appalled by this incredible sight, were now all panic-stricken. They accordingly decided to go in procession, barefoot and accompanied by priests, to Santa Maria della Scala, six miles from Messina. As they drew near the Virgin they all knelt as one, tearfully calling upon the help of God and the Virgin. They then entered the church with devout prayers, the priests chanting the psalm *miserere nostri Deus*, and laid hands upon a carving of the Mother of

---

found chantries, private chapels supported by one family or a small group of families. The great lords and millionaire gentry and merchants had always had private chapels. Along with the capability of having three hundred people for dinner in your household, it was the signal of conspicuous consumption of great wealth. . . .

Spiritually and intellectually, the century after the Black Death in England and elsewhere in northern Europe was marked by the rise of intense personal mysticism and separately by a privatist kind of bourgeois behavior in elaborate spiritual exercises. . . .

The other shift in late medieval religious sensibility was compulsive focus on the body of Christ. This inspired the elaboration of the Corpus Christi festivals and procession in the late medieval town and countryside. It drove the new fashion of taking the sacramental wafer as often as possible, instead of the old prescribed minimum communion of once a year. Eating Jesus in the Mass became the self-help mode of late medieval Christianity.

Norman F. Cantor, *In the Wake of the Plague: The Black Death and the World It Made.* New York: Free Press, 2001.

God, which had been placed there in ancient times and which they had chosen to take back to Messina, because they thought that upon its arrival the sight of it would drive out the demons from the city and deliver it from the mortality. Accordingly they chose a suitable priest to ride carrying the statue in his arms with due respect and so made their way back to the city with it.

As the holy Mother of God approached the city and saw it before her, all bloody with its sins, it was so hateful to her that she turned her back on it—she not only did not want to enter the city, but could not bear to look upon it. Therefore the earth gaped wide and the horse upon which the statue of the Mother of God was being carried became as fixed and immovable as a rock and could not be made to go either forwards or backwards. When the people of Messina saw these miracles they begged the Virgin, making their lamentations with sad sighs and frequent tears, that she would not take new revenge for their past sins. At their prayers the Virgin, the holy Bride of Christ, added her holy petitions to God to their humble prayers; whereupon the horse sets off again, the earth which had opened closes, and in a short time they had passed through the gate of the city into which the holy Mother of God had refused to enter. At last, accompanied by pious prayers to her, she made her entry into Santa Maria la Nuova, the main church of Messina, where the women of Messina smothered the statue with silk cloths and precious jewels.

But could not the holy Mother of God have remained in her church, she who totally refused to enter the city? Are we suggesting that she was carried unwillingly from her place? Indeed she could have remained there, since there is no power that could remove her—she to whom all mercy, all might, all goodness is granted by God's power—but it was so that the people, frantic with terror, might cleanse themselves completely of worldly allurements.

The Messinese Scatter Through Sicily

What more is there to say? The arrival of the statue profited nobody. On the contrary, the mortality raged even more, so that no one could help anyone else. Most of the citizens left Messina and scattered, some going to Calabria, others to various parts of Sicily, and especially to Catania. But what did this resort to flight avail them, given that the illness, already carried within them, was consuming their bodies? Of those who fled some collapsed in the roadway, in fields, on the shore, at sea, in the huts of Mascali, in woods, in ditches and in all manner of unlikely places. Those who made it to Catania breathed their last in lodgings—and they died in the city in such numbers that the Patriarch, in response to a demand by the citizens of Catania, ordered that no one from

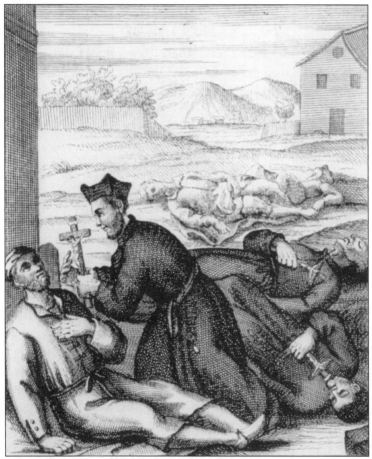

While tending to dying plague victims, priests often contracted the deadly disease and died shortly thereafter.

Messina should be buried within the city on pain of excommunication, but should instead be buried outside the city in good deep graves. What more is there to say? The Messinese were so loathed and feared that no man would speak with them, or be in their company, but hastily fled at the sight of them, holding his breath. And all the Catanians turned this into a sour joke, so that if anyone made to speak to someone that person would reply, in the vernacular, 'Don't talk to me if you're from Messina'. No one would give them shelter, so that they could not find houses in which to live, and unless other Messinese already established in the city gave them shelter secretly they were virtually without help.

And thus the Messinese were dispersed across the whole island. In going to Syracuse their illness infected the Syracusans so thoroughly that it was the death of a great many people. The regions around Sciacca and Trapani and the city of Agrigento also shared the pestilence with the Messinese in the same way—and especially Trapani, which has remained almost bereft of people. And what can we say about Catania, which has been delivered to oblivion? So strongly did the plague spring up there that not only the pustules commonly called *antrachi* but also a sort of tumour would erupt in various parts of the body—some on the chest, others on the legs, arms or throat. These tumours were at first the size of hazel nuts, and were accompanied by a marked stiffness and coldness. They so weakened and tormented the human body that at last the victim, unable to stay on his feet, had to take to his bed, by which stage he would be burning with a very high fever and suffering profound depression. These tumours grew to the size of a walnut and then to the size of a hen or goose egg, and their intense pain, and the accompanying putrefaction of humours, caused the victim to cough up blood, and this sputum, in passing from the infected lungs into the throat, corrupted the whole body. And it was from this corruption, and from the imperfection of the humours, that the victims died. The illness lasted three days; on the fourth day at the latest the victims went the way of all flesh.

The Catanians were well aware that the illness quickly proved fatal, and when they felt the depression and the cold stiffness coming over them their immediate priority was to make full confession of their sins to a priest and then make their wills. But the mortality was so great in the city that judges and notaries refused to go and draw up wills; and if they did visit a sick man they stood well away from him. Even priests were afraid to visit the sick for fear of death. And the mortality was so great that the judges and notaries were unable to meet the demand for wills, or the priests for hearing confession. Accordingly the Patriarch, concerned for the souls of the Catanians, bestowed upon every priest, however lowly, the same power to absolve sins which he enjoyed as bishop and patriarch. As a result, it is believed on the best authority that all those who died passed without fail safely to God.

Duke Giovanni, afraid of death and not wanting to come near cities or other settlements because of the infected air, ranged ceaselessly through wild and uninhabited places. And as he roamed here and there like a fugitive—now at *aqua mili* in the forest of Catania, now at a tower called *lu blancu* six miles from Catania, now at the church of San Salvatore *de blanchardu* in the forest of Catania—he came at last to a church or place called Sant'Andrea, newly built by him within the woods of Mascali, where, while he was living safe and sound, illness came upon him and he died. His body was buried in the main church of Catania, in the tomb where the former king Federico, his father, was buried. And this was in April 1348.

The mortality lasted from September more or less until the time of the duke's death. The mortality was so heavy that sex and age made no difference, but everyone died alike. . . . The Patriarch died in this mortality and was buried in the main church in Catania, may his soul rest in peace.

How to Survive the Plague

John of Burgundy

Upon the arrival of the Black Death, the fourteenth-century physicians of Europe found themselves completely at a loss. Bacteria and viruses were still unknown, and nobody realized that the disease was being transmitted among people and animals by the bite of infected fleas. The only certain prevention seemed to be complete isolation, as it was certain that people who came into contact with the sick were more likely to get the disease than those who held themselves aloof or escaped the affected cities altogether.

Nevertheless, many leading doctors did make an effort to apply the medicine they knew to this mysterious sickness. In 1365, John of Burgundy wrote one of the most thorough medical tracts concerning the Black Death. He theorized that the plague took the form of evil vapors which took root in the heart, liver, or brain, and that these vapors could be isolated and drawn out of the body by bleeding and by electuaries, medicinal preparations applied at the points of the skin where the disease manifested itself. Although these remedies were quite useless against a raging bacteria, their application may have given some relief to the sick in the form of boosting morale and a hope, however misplaced, of a cure.

Everything below the moon, the elements and the things compounded of the elements, is ruled by the things above, and the highest bodies are believed to give being, nature, substance, growth and death to everything below their

John of Burgundy, "The Treatise of John of Burgundy, 1365," translated and edited by Rosemary Horrox, *The Black Death*. Manchester, UK: Manchester University Press, 1994. Copyright © 1994 by Rosemary Horrox. Reproduced by permission of the publisher.

spheres. It was, therefore, by the influence of the heavenly bodies that the air was recently corrupted and made pestilential. I do not mean by this that the air is corrupted in its substance—because it is an uncompounded substance and that would be impossible—but it is corrupted by reason of evil vapours mixed with it. The result was a widespread epidemic, traces of which still remain in several places. Many people have been killed, especially those stuffed full of evil humours, for the cause of the mortality is not only the corruption of the air, but the abundance of corrupt humours within those who die of the disease. For as Galen [an ancient Greek physician, whom medieval doctors considered a paramount authority on medicine] says in the book of fevers, the body suffers no corruption unless the material of the body has a tendency towards it, and is in some way subject to the corruptive cause; for just as fire only takes hold on combustible material, so pestilential air does no harm to a body unless it finds a blemish where corruption can take hold. As a result, cleansed bodies, where the purgation of evil humours has not been neglected, remain healthy. Likewise those whose complexion is contrary to the immutable complexion of air remain healthy. For otherwise everybody would fall ill and die whenever the air is corrupted.

It follows that corrupt air generates different diseases in different people, depending on their different humours, because it always develops according to the predisposition of the matter it has entered. And therefore there are many masters of the art of medicine who are admirable scholars, well-versed in theories and hypotheses, but who are too little experienced in the practicalities and are entirely ignorant of astrology: a science vital to the physician. . . .

It is accordingly obvious that physic is of little effect without astrology, and as a result of a lack of advice many succumb to disease. And therefore I, John of Burgundy, otherwise known as Bearded John, citizen of Liège and practitioner of the art of medicine, although the least of physicians, produced a treatise at the beginning of this epidemic on the causes and nature of corrupt air, of which many people acquired copies. I also published a treatise on the difference between epidemic and other illness. Anyone who has copies will find many things in these treatises about lifestyle and cures— but not everything about cures. Because the epidemic is now newly returned, and will return again in future because it has not yet run its course, and because I pity the carnage among mankind and support the common good and desire the health of all, and have been moved by a wish to help, I intend, with

Taking Preventive Measures

In his book The Black Death, *historian Philip Ziegler lists a few of the many steps recommended by the medical experts of the time to prevent a case of the plague.*

There was general agreement . . . on the best kinds of preventive medicine. A fig or two with some rue and filberts taken before breakfast was a useful start to the day. Pills of aloes, myrrh and saffron were popular. One authority placed his confidence in ten-year-old treacle blended with some sixty elements, including chopped-up snakes, and mixed with good wine. Rhubarb and spikenard was a compound easier to manufacture and to swallow. Witchcraft joined herbalism in the works of Gentile of Foligno who recommended powdered emerald; a remedy so potent that, if a toad looked at it, its eyes would crack. Gentile also suggested etching on an amethyst the figure of a man bowing, girded with a serpent whose head he held in his right hand and whose tail in his left. To be fully operative the stone had first to be set in a gold ring.

Bleeding was generally held to be a useful preventive device; Ibn Khātimah, for instance, feeling that it could only be beneficial to lose up to eight pounds. Diet was important. Anything which quickly went bad in hot weather was to be avoided. So was fish from the infected waters of the sea. Meat should be roast rather than boiled. Eggs were authorised if eaten with vinegar but should never be taken hardboiled. Anyone trying to follow the advice of every expert would have been sadly perplexed. Ibn Khātimah approved

God's help, to set out more clearly in this schedule the prevention and cure of these illnesses, so that hardly anyone should have to resort to a physician but even simple folk can be their own physician, preserver, ruler and guide.

Concerning Prevention

First, you should avoid over-indulgence in food and drink, and also avoid baths and everything which might rarefy the

of fresh fruit and vegetables but no one else agreed. Gentile of Foligno recommended lettuce, the Faculty of Medicine at Paris forbade it. Ibn Khātimah had faith in egg plant, another expert deplored its use.

It was bad to sleep by day or directly after meals. Gentile believed that it was best to keep steady the heat of the liver by sleeping first on the right side and then on the left. To sleep on one's back was disastrous since this would cause a stream of superfluities to descend on the palate and nostrils. From thence these would flow back to the brain and submerge the memory.

Bad drove out bad and a school of thought maintained that to imbibe foul odours was a useful if not infallible protection. According to John Colle: 'Attendants who take care of latrines and those who serve in hospitals and other malodorous places are nearly all to be considered immune.' It was not unknown for apprehensive citizens of a plague-struck city to spend hours each day crouched over a latrine absorbing with relish the foetid smells.

A tranquil mind was one of the surer armours against infection. Ideally one should retreat to Boccaccio's enchanted glade, live beautifully, pass one's time in dalliance and in practising the art of conversation. But dalliance should not be carried too far: sex, like wrath, heated the members and disturbed the equilibrium. One's mind should be resolutely closed to the agonies of one's fellow men; sadness cooled the body, dulled the intelligence and deadened the spirit.

Philip Ziegler, *The Black Death*. New York: John Day, 1969.

body and open the pores, for the pores are the doorways through which poisonous air can enter, piercing the heart and corrupting the life force. Above all sexual intercourse should be avoided. You should eat little or no fruit, unless it is sour, and should consume easily-digested food and spiced wine diluted with water. Avoid mead [a popular fermented alcoholic drink] and everything else made with honey, and season food with strong vinegar. In cold or rainy weather you should light fires in your chamber and in foggy or windy weather you should inhale aromatics every morning before leaving home: ambergris, musk, rosemary and similar things if you are rich; zedoary, cloves, nutmeg, mace and similar things if you are poor. . . .

If, however, the epidemic occurs during hot weather it becomes necessary to adopt another regimen, and to eat cold things rather than hot and also to eat more sparingly than in cold weather. You should drink more than you eat, and take white wine with water. You should also use large amounts of vinegar and verjuice [a liquor made of the sour juice of crab apples and unripe fruits] in preparing food, but be sparing with hot substances such as pepper, galingale or grains of paradise. Before leaving home in the morning smell roses, violets, lilies, white and red sandalwood, musk or camphor if the weather is misty or the air quality bad. Take theriac [molasses] sparingly in hot weather, and not at all unless you are a phlegmatic or of a cold complexion. Sanguines and cholerics should not take theriac at all in hot weather, but should take pomegranates, oranges, lemons, or quinces, or an electuary [medicinal paste] made of the three types of sandalwood, or a cold electuary or similar. You should use cucumbers, fennel, borage, bugloss and spinach, and avoid garlic, onions, leeks and everything else which generates excessive heat, such as pepper or grains of paradise, although ginger, cinnamon, saffron, cummin and other temperate substances can be used. And if you should become extremely thirsty because of the hot weather, then drink cold water mixed with vinegar or barleywater regularly, for this is particularly beneficial to people of a cold and dry complexion and to thin people, and thirst should never be tolerated at such times.

If you should feel a motion of the blood like a fluttering or prickling, let blood from the nearest vein on the same side of the body, and the floor of the room in which you are lying should be sprinkled two or three times a day with cold water and vinegar, or with rose water if you can afford it. The pills of Rasis, if taken once a week, are an outstanding preventative and work for all complexions and in all seasons, but Avicenna [a medieval Arab physician] and others recommend that they should be taken on a full stomach. They loosen the bowels a little, but the corrupt humours are expelled gradually. They should be made as follows: take socotra aloes, saffron, myrrh and blend them in a syrup of fumitory. Anyone who adopts this regimen can be preserved, with God's help, from pestilence caused by corruption of the air.

Concerning the Cure of the Swelling

Now if anyone should contract epidemic disease for lack of a good regimen it is necessary to look at remedies and at how he should proceed, for these epidemic diseases take hold in twenty four hours and it is therefore vital to apply a remedy immediately. But first it should be understood that there are three principal members in the human body: the heart, the liver and the brain, and that each of these has its emunctory, where it expels its waste matter. Thus the armpits are the emunctories of the heart, the groin for the liver, and under the ears or beneath the tongue for the brain. Now it is necessary to know that it is the nature of poison to descend from the stomach, as is shown by the bite of a serpent or other venomous creature. And thus poisonous air, when it has been mixed with blood, immediately seeks the heart, the seat of nature, to attack it. The heart, sensing the injury, labours to defend itself, driving the poisoned blood to its emunctory. If then the venomous matter finds its way blocked, so that it cannot ascend back to the heart by some other path, it seeks another principal member, the liver, so that it can destroy that. The liver, fighting back, drives the resinous matter to its emunctory. In the same way it lays claim to the brain. By means of these events, which are signs to the physician, it is possible to tell where the poisonous matter is lurking and by what vein it ought to be drained.

For if the infected blood is driven to the armpits it can be deduced that the heart is oppressed and suffering, and so blood should be let immediately from the cardiac vein, but on the same side of the body, not the opposite side, for that would do double damage: firstly, the good and pure blood on the uncorrupted side would be drained away; secondly, the corrupt and poisoned blood would be thereby drawn to the healthy side of the body, with the result that the blood on both sides would become corrupted. What is worse, in the process the venomous blood would pass through the region of the heart and infect it, and thereby cause the rapid onset of illness. If, however, the patient feels prickings in the region of the liver, blood should be let immediately from the basilic vein of the right arm (that is the vein belonging to the liver, which is immediately below the vein belonging to the heart) or in the cephalic vein of the right hand, which is between the third and little fingers. . . .

When the blood has been extracted in this way, and the principal members purged, strengthen them with a cold electuary to offset any febrile cardiac inflammation. . . .

Diet in these illnesses should be as in the case of fevers, since the illness is always accompanied by fever. Therefore no meat should be eaten, except occasionally a small chicken poached in water and verjuice. Patients should eat small scaly fish, grilled on a gridiron with vinegar or verjuice, and soup of almonds, and drink barley water or small ale. If the patient demands wine, he should be given vinegar mixed with plenty of water. Occasionally, however, he can be given, to cheer him up, white wine diluted with plenty of water. . . .

Statement of the Times for Bloodletting

Certain lords have sought from me a schedule of what ought to be known to perform bleeding, and whether it should be done immediately or on the first or second day, and they are the people to whom I have addressed these things concerning the onset of illness.

I say that these pestilential illnesses have a short and sudden beginning and a rapid development, and therefore in these illnesses those who wish to work a cure ought not to delay, and bleeding, which is the beginning of the cure, should not be put off until the first or second day. On the contrary, if someone can be found to do it, blood should be taken from the vein going from the seat of the diseased matter (that is, in the place where morbidity has appeared) in the very hour in which the patient was seized by illness. And if the bleeding cannot be done within the hour, at least let it be done within six hours, and if that is not possible then do not let the patient eat or drink until the bleeding has been done. But do not by any means delay the bleeding for longer than twelve hours,

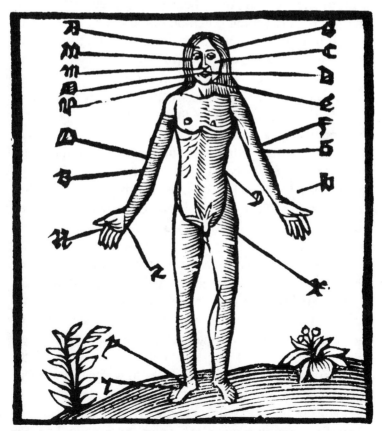

This picture is part of a bloodletting guide in a medieval reference manual. The lines leading to the body indicate the points from which blood is to be let.

for if it is done within twelve hours, while the poisonous matter is still moving about the body, it will certainly save the patient. But if it is delayed until the illness is established, and then done, it will certainly do no harm but there is no certainty that it will rescue the patient from danger, for by then the bad blood will be so clotted and thickened that it will be scarcely able to flow from the vein. If, after the phlebotomy, the poisonous matter spreads again, the bleeding should be repeated in the same vein or in another going from the seat of the diseased matter. Afterwards three or five spoonsful of the herbal water, made as above, should be administered.

And if not as much as that is available, let one spoonful be given morning and evening, and one spoonful should always be given after consumption of the electuary described above, whether by day (when it can be given at any hour) or by night. Or let the patient be given this confection, which strengthens the heart; expels harmful flatulence from it and quenches fever. Take conserves of violets, roses, bugloss, borage and oranges, powdered roses and sandalwood, cold tragacanth, an electuary of the three sandalwoods, powder to encourage moistness, a cold electuary, camphor and candied roses, mix them together without applying heat and place them in a box, and if the patient is of a hot complexion, or if the fever is intense, add six or seven grains of camphor. If the patient is rich and can afford it, pearls, gold leaf, pure silver, jacinths, emeralds, and the bone from the heart of a stag should be added. In the course of more than twenty four years of experience in places where the epidemic held sway it has been certainly and frequently demonstrated that such all electuary, together with the prescribed regimen, can save the patient from death. And many people have been cured by one bleeding alone, performed at the right time, without any other medicine. But where people delay bleeding beyond the development of the disease, it is doubtful whether it will lead to a cure or not. For while nature keeps the matter in motion, and the heart by its expulsive virtue drives the noisome and infected blood to its emunctory, phlebotomy should be performed because it helps nature, in that the extraction and evacuation of blood strengthens the expulsive virtue of the heart and diminishes the quantity of unhealthy matter, whereby nature is made more powerful against what remains and medicine becomes more efficacious.

I have never known anyone treated with this type of bleeding who has not escaped death, provided that he has looked after himself well and has received substances to strengthen his heart. As a result I make bold to say—not in criticism of past authorities, but out of long experience in the matter—that modern masters are more experienced in treating pestilential epidemic diseases than all the doctors and medical experts from Hippocrates downward. For none of them saw an epidemic reigning in their time, apart from Hippocrates in the city of *Craton* and that was short-lived. Nevertheless, he drew on what he had seen in his book on epidemics. However, Galen, Dioscorides, Rhazes 'Damascenus', Geber, Mesue, Copho, Constantine, Serapion, Avicenna, Algazel and all their successors never saw a general or long-lasting epidemic, or tested their cures by long experience; although they draw on the sayings of Hippocrates to discuss many things concerning epidemics. As a result, the masters of the present day are more practised in these diseases than their predecessors, for it is said, and with truth, that experience makes skill. Moved by piety and by pity for the destruction of men, I have accordingly compiled this compendium and have specified and set out the veins to bleed in these epidemic diseases, so that anyone may be his own physician. And because these illness run their course very quickly, and the poisonous matter rages through the body, let the bleeding be done without delay according to my advice, for in many cases delay brings danger.

I have composed and compiled this work not for money but for prayers, and so let anyone who has recovered from the disease pray strongly for me to our Lord God, to whom be the praise and glory throughout the whole world for ever and ever, amen.

Here ends the valuable treatise of Master John of Burgundy against epidemic disease.

Chapter 4

Social and Economic Impact of the Plague

Chapter Preface

By the time the plague had subsided, about one-third of Europe's population had died. In many ways, the Black Death was an important turning point in the history of Europe, where economics, politics, and society would never be the same. It marked the beginning of the end of the medieval period and the start of a social transformation of the continent.

The most important effects were economic. Europe had lost millions of productive laborers. Crops went unplanted and unharvested, and vast tracts of farmland returned to wilderness. The food supply dwindled, but so did the demand for food and other goods. Prices fell, and the sudden shortage of workers raised the value of work. The plague also loosened the feudal bonds that tied peasants to the land and to the aristocratic class of landowners. With better opportunities beckoning in the cities, rural peasants flooded the towns. They joined craft guilds and hired out their skills to whoever could pay them.

The undermining of the feudal system weakened the dominance of landowners over society. No longer able to rule their domains as semi-independent manorial lords, the European nobility saw their power wane and that of the kings rise. The crowned heads of Europe were able to consolidate their power, and the first great European nation-states began to emerge.

The plague also caused a questioning of the religious hierarchy. As far as the people could see, the supplications of priests and bishops to God had done little to stem the awful tide. The clergy, who presided at the most important events in one's life, lost some of the common people's fearful respect. Although there had been widespread dissent and criticism of the practices of the church, the restlessness now became widespread. Within a few decades, the first stirrings of a break with the church hierarchy would occur, ultimately leading to the Protestant Reformation of the sixteenth century.

In many cases, these effects would take centuries to be assimilated. Although the plague continued in the form of sporadic outbreaks, its social effects would continue to ripple through Europe.

Blaming the Jews for the Plague

Anonymous

In medieval times, the Jews of Europe were widely suspected of crimes against the dominant Christian society. Where they were tolerated at all, Jewish citizens were restricted to certain neighborhoods (known as "ghettos" after the Jewish quarter in Venice). They were forbidden to hold certain jobs, to educate themselves in schools, fight in armies, or enlist in the service of monarchs. Thus segregated from the mainstream, the Jews made an easy target for accusations that they had deliberately brought the plague down on their Christian neighbors.

The fact that Jews died of the plague as readily as did non-Jews did not convince their accusers. By the thousands, Jews were rounded up, tortured on a stretching rack or otherwise in order to exact "confessions" of instigating or perpetuating the Black Death. Two such confessions, those of men named Balavignus and Manssiono, were preserved for history in a legal document of September 15, 1348, from the city of Neustadt, Germany. After surviving the rack and signing such a confession, the accused were no doubt executed, possibly in one of the mass burnings that occurred commonly during the Black Death.

The Confession of Balavignus

Balavignus, a Jewish physician, inhabitant of Thonon, was arrested at Chillon in consequence of being found in the neighbourhood. He was put for a short time to the rack, and

J.F.C. Hecker, *The Epidemics of the Middle Ages*, translated by B.G. Babington. London: Trubner and Company, 1859.

on being taken down, confessed, after much hesitation, that, about ten weeks before, the Rabbi Jacob of Toledo, who, because of a citation, had resided at Chamberi since Easter, sent him, by a Jewish boy, some poison in the mummy of an egg: it was a powder sewed up in a thin leathern pouch accompanied by a letter, commanding him on penalty of excommunication, and by his required obedience to the law, to throw this poison into the larger and more frequented wells of the town of Thonon, to poison those who drew water there. He was further enjoined not to communicate the circumstance to any person whatever, under the same penalty. In conformity with this command of the Jewish rabbis and doctors of the law, he, Balavignus, distributed the poison in several places, and acknowledged having one evening placed a certain portion under a stone in a spring on the shore at Thonon. He further confessed that the said boy brought various letters of a similar import, addressed to others of his nation, and particularly specified some directed severally to Mossoiet, Banditon, and Samoleto of Neustadt; to Musseo Abramo and Aquetus of Montreantz, Jews residing at Thurn in Vivey; to Benetonus and his son at St. Moritz; to Vivianus Jacobus, Aquetus and Sonetus, Jews at Aquani.—Several letters of a like nature were sent to Abram and Musset, Jews at Moncheoli; and the boy told him that he had taken many others to different and distant places, but he did not recollect to whom they were addressed. Balavignus further confessed that, after having put the poison into the spring at Thonon, he had positively forbidden his wife and children to drink the water, but had not thought fit to assign a reason. He avowed the truth of this statement, and, in the presence of several credible witnesses, swore by his Law, and the Five Books of Moses, to every item of his deposition.

On the day following, Balavignus, voluntarily and without torture, ratified the above confession verbatim before many persons of character, and, of his own accord, acknowledged that, on returning one day from Tour near Vivey, he had thrown into a well below Mustruez, namely, that of La Conerayde, a quantity of the poison tied up in a

The Black Death and the Jews of Europe

In The Illustrated History of the Jewish People, *Nicholas de Lange describes the anti-Jewish hysteria that gripped Europe during the Black Death, a time when the segregated Jews made a convenient scapegoat for the mysterious epidemic.*

Anti-Jewish violence during the Black Death was unprecedented in its geographical extent, the number of Jews who lost their lives and the grave danger to the continued existence of the Jewish centers of Europe. It was the worst calamity to befall the Jews of Europe until the Holocaust. The massacres began in the south of France, proceeding from there westward to Spain and northward to France and Germany. In dread of the plague, people sought human agents for the disease, and the Jews were accused of poisoning wells—an allegation that made its first appearance in Savoy in the summer of 1348 and spread from there to the German Reich [Holy Roman Empire]. It was held that the Jews had launched a worldwide conspiracy to destroy Christian Europe. Although the libel was disbelieved by intellectuals, and even the pope denied its truth, the uneducated masses were convinced of its veracity and accordingly "defended" themselves by particularly savage assaults. . . .

Although the immediate motive for the attacks was the accusation of well poisoning, modern scholarship has shown that the reasons were more complex. In some places, those responsible for the violence were the leading burghers, who were eager to seize Jewish property and to that end manipulated the popular hatred. . . . The economic crisis of the fourteenth century, escalating insecurity and fear of famine, plagues and other natural calamities all instilled in the common people of Europe feelings of xenophobia and endowed all strangers with a diabolical image.

Nicholas de Lange, ed., *The Illustrated History of the Jewish People.* New York: Harcourt Brace, 1997.

rag, given to him for the purpose by Aquetus of Montreantz, an inhabitant of the said Tour: that he had acquainted Manssiono, and his son Delosaz, residents of Neustadt, with the circumstance of his having done so, and advertised them not to drink of the water. He described the colour of the poison as being red and black.

On the nineteenth day of September, the above-named Balavignus confessed, without torture, that about three weeks after Whitsuntide, a Jew named Mussus told him that he had thrown poison into the well, in the custom-house of that place, the property of the Borneller family; and that he no longer drank the water of this well, but that of the lake. He further deposed that Mussus informed him that he had also laid some of the poison under the stones in the custom-house at Chillon. Search was accordingly made in this well, and the poison found: some of it was given to a Jew by way of trial, and he died in consequence. He also stated that the rabbis had ordered him and other Jews to refrain from drinking of the water for nine days after the poison was infused into it; and immediately on having poisoned the waters, he communicated the circumstance to the other Jews. He, Balavignus, confessed that about two months previously, being at Evian, he had some conversation on the subject with a Jew called Jacob, and among other things, asked him whether he also had received writings and poison, and was answered in the affirmative; he then questioned him whether he had obeyed the command, and Jacob replied that he had not, but had given the poison to Savetus, a Jew, who had thrown it into the well de Morer at Evian. Jacob also desired him, Balavignus, to execute the command imposed on him with due caution. He confessed that Aquetus of Montreantz had informed him that he had thrown some of the poison into the well above Tour, the water of which he sometimes drank. He confessed that Samolet had told him that he had laid the poison which he had received in a well, which, however, he refused to name to him. Balavignus, as a physician, further deposed that a person infected by such poison coming in contact with another while in a state of perspiration, infection would be the almost inevitable result; as might also happen from the breath of an infected person. This fact he believed to be correct, and was confirmed in his opinion by the attestation of many experienced physicians. He also declared that none of his community could exculpate themselves from this accusation, as the plot was communicated to all; and that all were guilty of the above charges. Balavignus was conveyed over the lake from Chillon to Clarens, to point out the well into which he confessed having thrown the powder. On landing, he was conducted to the spot; and, having seen the well, acknowledged that to be the place, saying, "This is the well into which I put the poison." The well was examined in his presence, and the linen cloth in which the poison had been wrapped was found in the wastepipe by a notary-public named Heinrich Gerhard, in the presence of many persons, and was shown to the said Jew. He acknowledged this to be the linen which had contained the poison, which he described as being of two colours, red and black, but said that he had thrown it into the open well. The linen cloth was taken away and is preserved.

Balavignus, in conclusion, attests the truth of all and everything as above related. He believes this poison to contain a portion of the basilisk, because he had heard, and felt assured, that the above poison could not be prepared without it. . . .

The Confession of Manssiono

Manssiono, Jew of Neustadt, was put upon the rack on the fifteenth day of the same month, but refused to admit the above charge, protesting his entire ignorance of the whole matter; but the day following, he, voluntarily and without any torture, confessed, in the presence of many persons, that he came from Mancheolo one day in last Whitsun-week, in company with a Jew named Provenzal, and, on reaching the well of Chabloz Crüez between Vyona and Mura, the latter said, "You must put some of the poison which I will give you into that well, or woe betide you!" He therefore took a portion of the powder about the bigness of a nut, and did as he was directed. He believed that the Jews in the neighbourhood of Evian had convened a council among themselves relative to this plot, before Whitsuntide. He further said that Balavignus had informed him of his having poisoned the well de la Conerayde below Mustruez. He also affirmed his conviction of the culpability of the Jews in this affair, stating that they were fully acquainted with all the particulars, and guilty of the alleged crime.

On the third day of the October following, Manssiono was brought before the commissioners, and did not in the least vary from his former deposition, or deny having put the poison into the said wells.

The above-named Jews, prior to their execution, solemnly swore by their Law to the truth of their several depositions, and declared that all Jews whatsoever, from seven years old and upwards, could not be exempted from the charge of guilt, as all of them were acquainted with the plot, and more or less participators in the crime.

The Flagellants Do Penance

Hugo von Reutlingen

In the wake of the Black Death, the society of medieval
Europe underwent a wrenching self-examination, searching
for causes as well as some means to prevent the plague from
ever occurring again. Since the medical causes of the plague
were unknown, people looked for answers elsewhere, particularly in the realm of the spiritual life. Priests and clergymen
delivered sermons to inspire the faithful to a better life, while
thousands of people joined religious orders to dedicate themselves completely to the service of God. To do penance for
the sins of the world, and to head off future visitations of the
plague, the sect of flagellants arose in 1349. Members wandered in large groups along the roads of Europe, whipping
and scourging themselves in public squares in expiation for
the sins of the world.

In the following chronicle, the German chronicler Hugo
von Reutlingen describes the flagellants as they practiced
their beliefs. Although many who witnessed these public
scourgings admired the flagellants, the church saw them as
dangerous and seditious, and officially condemned them.
Eventually, as medieval society gradually returned to normal,
the sect faded away, but not without leaving a vivid memory
of their extreme practices.

L et me relate to you in proper detail what happened on
the earth then, in those ever memorable days, although

Hugo von Reutlingen, "The Flagellant Chronicle of Hugo von Reutlingen: Statutes of the
Flagellants," *The Black Death: A Chronicle of the Plague*, translated by C.H. Clarke,
edited by Johannes Nohl. London: George Allen and Unwin, 1926.

the events and the times of which I write are doubtless known to you. At that time the flagellants were wandering about the country in crowds on all the roads and paths, cruelly martyrising their bodies themselves with blows of the cruel knots which they had tied in their scourges [whips], for in every scourge the knots were tied threefold; such was the order. All who joined the movement placed themselves under the sign of the cross, because all are acceptable to the Virgin's Son who without feign piously make the sign of the cross, as prescribed by the Scriptures or those who wear it. You would see a few crosses sewn on the cloaks, in the same way the brethren must provide, too, for the hats they wore. Cloaks and overclothing of this kind were worn by all of them, but their underclothing was not marked with the cross. When food was brought them they covered their heads with their hats. And it must never be omitted when the scourging goes round, as also when eating, that they should have the cross before their eyes. . . .

Flagellant Rituals

Two pieces of iron, with sharpened upper end passing through the knots, beat the backs of the penitents and caused a ring of four-cornered wounds. Priest and landgrave, knight and knave, here are all companions—even the masters of different schools are in close agreement, citizens, students, vagrants, and peasants. For thirty-four days the pilgrims spend the night in different quarters, changing each night, because for this same number of years Christ walked upon earth, dwelling in many and often poor shelters. But the last day they count only as half; each one turns his steps homewards before it is ended. But still it is counted as a full day like the others, for Christ, too, shortened His last year on earth, rising to His Eternal Kingdom, ascending to heaven. Once during the night and twice in the daytime they tortured themselves with cruel blows, while the singing of hymns sounded with astonishing cadence and, marching in a circle, they threw themselves down to the ground and in such a manner as to form a cross. This they used to do six times a day, and they remained so long as one might say a few paternosters. When they arose there was further singing and scourging, which pained them more than that which had gone before; whilst once more they wound round in a circle, as they were ordered; their feet being bare, from the navel to the ankle, they were clad with cloth of poor quality to conceal what shame demands that we should hide; but their trunks, except their heads, they had bare. Once every night each one beat himself for the space of time during which he could say seven paternosters as quickly as he could, and during the scourging he had to cover his head with his hat and also during the night. Before sitting down to a meal each had to say two paternosters, and another three when the meal was finished. But here there was no master receiving water from his servant to wash his hands, when required in a basin; but for the common use of all there stood on the ground a vessel dripping with water for the washing of hands. It was strictly forbidden to the brethren to ask for a bath at any time or to wash their heads. No one was allowed to speak to a woman, and just as little to have his beard shorn, except in special cases when the master gave permission to some brother. Nor would anyone have dared to wear freshly washed clothes before the time for changing had duly come. They were strict in their observance of Sunday; they never marched separately, but at night they occupied separate quarters—there where yesterday one slept the next day another came. Besides, they did not sleep in beds, but their bed was straw with a light cloth spread over it—but they were permitted to place a cushion under their heads. After every five days they fasted, and on fast days they scourged themselves three times, all being assembled, and threw themselves nine times on the ground, three times at each scourging.

Rules of the Order

In regard to the number of flagellants it should be observed that they were seldom found in the same number; sometimes a thousand together were assembled in the neighbourhood of some town, frequently they marched in quite a small company, or, still more frequently, they dispersed in different groups, if they had assembled in too great numbers and wished to remain welcome guests among the lay population.

The Travels of the Penitents

The medieval French chronicler Jean Froissart described the many miseries of the Black Death and the Hundred Years War in his work. In the following passage, the flagellants wander through the countryside, inspiring acts of devotion and penitence and striking great fear in the Jewish communities of the towns they visited.

In the Year of Grace 1349, the penitents went about, coming first out of Germany. They were men who did public penance and scourged themselves with whips of hard knotted leather with little iron spikes. Some made themselves bleed very badly between the shoulders and some foolish women had cloths ready to catch the blood and smear it on their eyes, saying that it was miraculous blood. While they were doing penance, they sang very mournful songs about the nativity and passion of Our Lord.

The object of this penance was to entreat God to put a stop to the mortality, for in that time of death there was an epidemic of plague. People died suddenly and at least a third of all the people in the world died then. The penitents of whom I am speaking went in companies from town to town and from city to city and wore long felt hoods on their heads, each company with its own colour. Their rules forbade them to sleep more than one night in each town and the length of their goings-out was fixed by the thirty-three and a half years which Jesus Christ spent on earth, as the Holy Scriptures tell us; each of their companies went about for thirty-three and a half days, and then they returned to the towns or castles from which they had come. They spent very little money on their journeys, because the good people of the towns which they visited asked them to dinner and supper. They slept only on straw, unless illness forced them to do otherwise. When they entered a house in which they were

And although among them were many wise, sensible men, swindlers and madmen had joined their ranks, people ripe for the hangman's rope, as they were teeming with lies, and they often annoyed the clergy and their own companions

---

to dine or sup, they kneeled down humbly on the threshold and said three paternosters and three *Ave Marias*, and did the same when they left. . . .

Their rules contained some quite reasonable and acceptable things which agreed with such natural human inclinations as to journey about and do penance, but they did not enter the Kingdom of France because Pope Innocent, who was at Avignon at that time with his cardinals, considered the practice and opposed it very strongly, declaring in condemnation of the penitents that public penance inflicted by oneself was neither right nor lawful. They were excommunicated for doing it, and especially those clergy who went with them. A number of priests, canons and chaplains who supported them were deprived of their benefices. Any who wished for absolution had to go to Avignon to get it. So this movement was broken up and came to nothing when it was seen that the Pope and the King of France were against them, and they did not go beyond Hainault. If they had gone to Cambrai or Saint-Quentin, the gates would have been shut in their faces.

As soon as the penitents appeared and the news of them spread round, the sect of the Jews contemplated and feared their own destruction, for they had a prophecy made over two hundred years earlier which said in cryptic language: 'Knights will come bearing links of iron who will be very cruel, but they will have no leaders and their power and their works will not extend beyond the Empire of Germany. But when they come, we shall all be destroyed.' Their prophecy came true, for in those days all the Jews were indeed destroyed, though more in one country than in another. The Pope, and the Kings of [the Spanish realms of] Castile, Aragon and Navarre, accepted great numbers of them and laid them under tribute beneath them.

Geoffrey Brereton, ed. and trans., *Chronicles*. New York: Penguin, 1968.

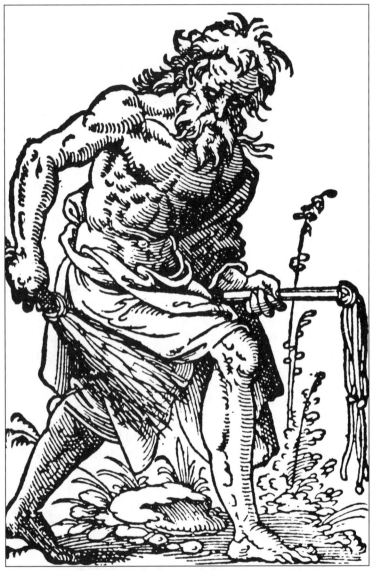

Believing that the plague was punishment for man's sins, the flagellants performed self-castigating rituals with the hope of appeasing God.

who were endeavouring to spread what is good and to avoid what is bad.

Further, all who had become brethren in this scourging fraternity had to fulfil some special duties, which we do not enumerate, all for the sake of brevity. He who went to the privy had to lay aside all clothing marked with the cross, which otherwise he must always wear. No brother was admitted without confession; anyone whom he had hurt by words, to him he must give full satisfaction; if he did not do this, whatever his rank, he was regarded as spurned by Christ and still in the toils of sin. Nor was anyone permitted to enter a house, to whomsoever it might belong, till invited by the master to enter as a guest, even if he wished to buy what he considered necessary. If no one invited them to their houses, they remained outside in the fields, or they stood in the fields till someone should let them in and give them the necessities of life and a night's lodging. They appointed masters over themselves to the number of two, sometimes only one, whose orders they observed strictly in every respect. Flags covered with crosses waved in the processions of the flagellants. Two by two, as if brothers of one family, they marched to the singing of hymns like students when on their way (they all had a common goal) to the place of scourging. The sound of bells mingles solemnly with their hymns as the procession passes through the town gate accompanied by the crowd, eager either to gaze at the wounds torn by the terrible scourges or to pray to the Lord, Who suffered on the Cross, in their hearts not to continue to destroy the people by the sudden death of the plague, to grant mercy to the dead and peace to the living till at the end of their life's course they laud and praise Him in heaven on high.

The Fate of the Sect

It is true that in many places abuses crept in; laity, all kinds of people, united together in swarms—indeed, even women were seen, and daily the people went out to see them without reflection. Who can tell what ultimately became of this rabble? Therefore I make no attempt; perhaps later, if God preserves my life, I may be able to narrate their fate. But now I will end and turn aside from the flagellants to whom the people still used to throng. Some bishops, princes, and lords united and issued severe commands supported by threats of hard measures; these together with snow, frost and mist, and the impending Holy Year, ultimately put an end to the wandering companies of brethren who found the means of torturing themselves so cruelly by their terrible scourging.

Their behaviour was obnoxious to the real, true clergy on account of lying legend and insipid doctrines. They even proclaimed that on a marble tablet above the altar of St. Peter at Jerusalem the true doctrine of belief was inscribed, whereas no such tablet ever existed there. The various hymns of the brethren also contained a multitude of foolish things and doctrines which might frequently be heard from them, but by many in their honest simplicity were not recognised as such. Some good there certainly was at the bottom of the fraternity; only thus is their great success and the high respect they enjoyed to be explained. Let anyone who knows more than he has read here reveal it!

Poisoning Rumors Incite Lynch Mobs

Heinrich Seuse

The plague brought fear as well as deep suspicion, as the people of Europe searched for the culprits who they believed had brought the disease in their midst. Oftentimes, traveling strangers were accused of poisoning wells or food supplies, and in these dangerous moments they had some fast explaining to do in order to save their own lives.

Just such a dangerous moment occurred to the German mystic Heinrich Seuse (Henry Suso). While traveling with a companion in the Rhineland, Seuse found himself the target of a lynch mob—inspired by an accusation made by his own companion. In the following autobiographical account, in which Seuse refers to himself in the third person as the "Servant," only the intercession of a kindly priest saves him from being run through with a pike.

Once, when he was about to set out on a journey, a companion was given to him, a lay brother, who was mentally unbalanced. He was reluctant to take him with him, for he recollected what trials he had suffered from his companions in the past. Yet finally he agreed, and took him with him.

Now it happened that they entered a village before breakfast. That day there was a fair, and all kinds of people had come to it. It had been raining, and his companion was wet through; he entered a house and went up to the fire, saying that he could go no further. He told the Servant to do his

Henry Suso, *The Life of the Servant*, translated by J.M. Clark. London: Clarke Company, Ltd, 1983. Copyright © 1952 by J.M. Clark. Reproduced by permission of the publisher.

business without him and said he would wait for him there.

Scarcely had the friar left the house, when his companion got up and sat at the table, joining some rough fellows and traders who had come to the fair. They saw that the wine had gone to his head; so when he got up and stood in the doorway, gaping at them, they seized him and said that he had stolen a cheese from them. While these wicked men were brutally ill-treating him, four or five soldiers came up and attacked him, and said that the evil monk was a poisoner of wells. For it was at this time that there were great rumours of poisoning abroad. So they seized him, and made such a commotion that many men ran up to the place.

A False Accusation

When the lay brother saw how things stood, and that he was a prisoner, he wanted to escape, so he turned round and cried out to them: 'Stop a while, stand still; let me say what I have to say, and I will tell you how it happened, for it is, alas, a sad story!' They stopped, and all listened. He began and said, 'Look and you will all see for yourselves that I am a fool and an ignorant man, and no one pays any attention to me. But my companion is a wise and experienced man. His Order has entrusted to him a bag of poison to sink in the wells, here and there in the country as far as Alsace, whither he is now bound. Everywhere he goes he will defile everything with deadly poison. See to it that you get him soon, or he will commit crimes that no one can ever undo. He has just taken out a little bag, and he has thrown it into the village well, so that all those who come to the fair, and drink out of the well, will be poisoned. That is why I stayed here, and would not go out, because I do not like it. And as a proof that I am telling the truth, you should know that he has a large sack, which is full of these bags of poison and with the gold pieces, that he and his Order have got from the Jews to pay him for committing these crimes.'

When the wild ruffians who had gathered round heard these words, they raged and cried with a loud voice: 'Come along, away with the murderer before he escapes!' One grasped his pike, another his axe, and each took any weapon he could find, and they ran with wild ferocious gestures. They broke open houses and monasteries, searching every place where they thought they might find him, thrusting their naked swords through bedding and straw, so that the whole fair came running along. People from other towns also came up, honourable men who knew the Servant. When they heard his name mentioned, they came forward and persuaded the mob that they were doing him an injustice, that he was a very pious man, who was incapable of committing such a crime. Not finding him, they finally desisted in their search, and took his companion to the judge as a prisoner. The latter ordered him to be locked up in a cell.

This went on until daybreak. The Servant knew nothing of these disturbances. When he thought it time to break his fast, and he hoped his companion had got dry before the fire, he entered the inn to have a meal. But when he entered the tavern, they began to tell him the whole story of what had happened. He ran forthwith in great alarm to the house where his companion and the judge were, and begged for his companion to be liberated. But the judge said this could not be done: he intended to commit him to prison for his crime. This was sad and doleful news for the Servant, who ran hither and thither to get help. But he could not find anyone who would help him. After carrying on his efforts with great shame and grief, he finally procured the man's release by payment of a heavy fine.

The Villagers Give Chase

He now thought his troubles were at an end, but they were only just beginning. For when, with pain and loss, he had escaped from the authorities, he fell into danger of his life. For, as he was leaving the judge, about the time of vespers, the rumour had spread among the common people and young boys that he was a poisoner. They denounced him as a murderer, so that he did not dare to leave the town. They pointed at him, and said: 'Look, fellows, that is the poisoner! He has kept out of our way all day; he must be put to death! His money won't help him with us, as it did with the judge!' When he tried to escape down the village, they cried out all the louder after him. Some said, 'We will drown him in the Rhine,' for this river flowed past the village. Others cried, 'No, the unclean murderer will pollute all the water; we should burn him alive.'

A huge peasant with a sooty jacket grabbed a pike, pushed between the others and cried, 'Listen to me, gentlemen all! We cannot inflict any more shameful death on the wicked heretic than this: I will thrust this long pike through him, as one does to a venomous toad that one impales. Just let me stick this pike through the naked body of this poisoner. I will lift him up from behind and fix him fast in this fence, and take care that he does not fall. Let his unclean corpse dry in the wind, so that all the people that pass to and fro will have a sight of the murderer, and will curse him after his shameful death, and that he may be all the more accursed both in this world and the next. For the vile scoundrel has well deserved it.'

The wretched Servant heard all this with bitter fear, groaning deeply, and the large tears ran down his face. All those who stood round in a circle, and saw him in his anguish, wept bitterly, and some beat their breasts with compassion, and struck their hands together over their heads. But no one dared to speak, fearing the dreadful rabble would attack them also. At nightfall, he went to and fro, begging with tears that for God's sake someone would have mercy and give him lodging. But he was cruelly driven away. Some kind women would gladly have given him shelter, but they did not dare to do so.

The wretched sufferer was thus in peril of his life, and all human help had deserted him, as everyone was just waiting to see them attack him and kill him. He fell down in anguish and fear of death in front of a fence, raised his wretched swollen eyes to the heavenly Father, saying: 'Alas, Father of all mercies, when wilt thou come to my aid today in my great distress? Alas, merciful heart, why hast Thou forgotten thy mercy to me? Alas, Father, alas, faithful, mild Father, help me, wretched man, in this great misery! I cannot take counsel with my own heart, since it is dead already, whether it would be more tolerable to drown, or to be burnt alive, or to die at the stake, yet I must suffer one of these deaths. I commend to Thee today my wretched spirit. Have mercy on me in the face of the miserable death that threatens me: they are near me who would destroy me.' This sorrowful lament came to the ears of a priest, who ran vigorously to him, dragged him out of their hands, took him to his house and kept him overnight, so that no harm came to him. Early the next morning he helped him to escape from all his troubles.

The Devastation of the English Clergy

William Dene

In the following account of 1349, the English monk William
Dene of Rochester describes how the plague ravaged the
church, carrying away entire households and leaving many
parishes completely bereft of churchmen (since the close
quarters in which monks and nuns lived made it easy for the
plague to travel from one victim to the next). Dene goes on to
describe the effect on English laborers, who found their numbers scarce and their services in high demand, and the general
greed and lawlessness that gripped the country as people died
by the thousands.

A plague such as never before had been heard of, . . . ravaged England in this year. The Bishop of Rochester, out
of his small household lost four priests, five gentlemen, ten
serving men, seven young clerks, and six pages, so that not a
soul remained who might serve him in any office. At Malling
(a Benedictine nunnery) he blessed two abbesses, and both
quickly died, and there were left there only four professed
nuns and four novices. To one of these the Bishop committed
the charge of the temporals, to another that of the spirituals,
because no proper person for abbess could be found.

The whole of this time . . . the Bishop of Rochester remained at Halling and Trotterscliff, and he conferred orders
in both places at certain intervals. Alas, for our sorrow! this
mortality swept away so vast a multitude of both sexes that

Francis Aidan Gasquet, *The Black Death of 1348 and 1349*. London: George Bell and
Sons, 1908.

none could be found to carry the corpses to the grave. Men and women bore their own offspring on their shoulders to the church and cast them into a common pit. From these there proceeded so great a stench that hardly anyone dared to cross the cemeteries. . . .

In this pestilence many chaplains and paid clerics refused to serve, except at excessive salaries. The Bishop of Rochester, by a mandate addressed to the archdeacon of Rochester, on the 27th of June, 1349, orders all these, on pain of suspension, to serve such cures [positions] . . . and some priests and clerics refuse livings [homes], now vacant in law and fact . . . "because they are slenderly provided for; and some, having poor livings, which they had long ago obtained, are now unwilling to keep them, because their stipend, on account of the death of their parishioners, is so notoriously diminished that they cannot get a living and bear the burden of their cure. It has accordingly happened that parishes have remained unserved for a long time, and the cure attached to them has been abandoned, to the great danger of souls. We, desiring to remedy this as soon as possible, by the present letters permit and grant special leave to all rectors and vicars of our city and diocese instituted, or hereafter to be instituted, to such slender benefices as do not produce a true revenue of ten marks sterling a year, to receive during their poverty an anniversary mass, or such a number of masses as may bring their stipends to this annual sum.". . .

So great was the deficiency of labourers and workmen of every kind in those days that more than a third of the land over the whole kingdom remained uncultivated. The labourers and skilled workmen were imbued with such a spirit of rebellion that neither king, law, nor justice could curb them. The whole people for the greater part ever became more depraved, more prone to every vice, and more inclined than before to evil and wickedness, not thinking of death, nor of the past plague, nor of their own salvation. . . . And priests, little weighing the sacrifice of a contrite spirit, betook themselves to places where they could get larger stipends than in their own benefices. On which account many benefices re-

Laymen Perform the Sacraments

So many clergymen died of the plague that the church was hard-pressed to replace its members. In January 1349, Ralph of Shrewsbury, the bishop of Bath and Wells, sent the following letter to priests working within his parish to announce that laymen may perform the sacraments.

The contagious pestilence of the present day, which is spreading far and wide, has left many parish churches and other livings in our diocese without parson or priest to care for their parishioners. Since no priests can be found who are willing, whether out of zeal and devotion or in exchange for a stipend, to take on the pastoral care of these aforesaid places, nor to visit the sick and administer to them the Sacraments of the Church (perhaps for fear of infection and contagion), we understand that many people are dying without the Sacrament of Penance. These people have no idea what recourses are open to them in such a case of need and believe that, whatever the straits they may be in, no confession of their sins is useful or meritorious unless it is made to a duly ordained priest. We, therefore, wishing, as is our duty, to provide for the salvation of souls and to bring back from their paths of error those who have wandered, do strictly enjoin and command, on the oath of obedience that you have sworn to us, you, the rectors, vicars and parish priests in all your churches, and you, the deans elsewhere in your deaneries where the comfort of a priest is denied the people, that, ei-

mained unserved, whose holders would not be stayed by the rule of their Ordinary. Thus, day by day, the dangers to soul both in clergy and in people multiplied.

Throughout the whole of that winter and spring the Bishop of Rochester, an old and decrepit man, remained at Trotterscliff, saddened and grieving over the sudden change of the age. And in every manor of the Bishopric buildings and walls fell to ruins, and that year there was hardly a manor which returned [earned] a hundred pounds. In the monastery of Rochester, also, there was such a scarcity of ther yourselves or through some other person you should at once publicly command and persuade all men, in particular those who are now sick or should fall sick in the future, that, if they are on the point of death and can not secure the services of a priest, then they should make confession to each other, as is permitted in the teaching of the Apostles, whether to a layman or, if no man is present, then even to a woman. We urge you, by these present letters, in the bowels of Jesus Christ, to do this . . . And, in case anyone might fear that a lay confessor would make public the confessions which they heard and, for this reason, might hesitate to confess himself to such a person even in time of need, you should announce to all in general and, in particular, to those who might hear confessions in this way, that they are bound by the laws of the Church to conceal and keep secret such confessions and that they are prohibited by sacred canonical decrees from betraying such confessions by word, sign, or any other means, except at the wish of those who have made such confession. If they break this law then they should know that they commit a most grievous sin and, in so doing, incur the wrath of Almighty God and of the whole Church. . . .

The Sacrament of the Eucharist, when no priest is available, may be administered by a deacon. If, however, there is no priest to administer the Sacrament of Extreme Unction, then, as in other matters, faith must suffice.

Philip Ziegler, *The Black Death.* New York: John Day, 1969.

provisions that the community were troubled with great want of food; so much so that the monks were obliged to grind their own bread.

Ordinances for a Time of Plague

The Elders of Pistoia

Tuscany, a region of northern Italy, was one of the wealthiest and most industrialized areas of fourteenth-century Europe. Tuscan towns were governed by elected councils, and presided over by a *podesta*, usually an outsider with no business or family connections to the city he governed and who served a short term. The members of the city governments openly debated all issues confronting them and were free to pass ordinances in a time of emergency. Thus free of the whims and tyranny of a monarch or dictator, the cities of Tuscany were as well-equipped to deal with the Black Death as any in Europe.

In the spring of 1348, while the Black Death approached, the *anziani*, or elders, of the city of Pistoia promulgated the following ordinances to deal with the disease. The ordinances attempted to keep out plague-stricken people and possibly infected material, to mandate the healthiest way of disposing of the dead, and to segregate as much as possible plague-stricken families of the city from the still-healthy population. Despite these measures, which were medically sound for the time, Pistoia lost approximately one-fourth of its population to the plague.

In the name of Christ Amen. Herein are written certain ordinances and provisions made and agreed upon by certain wise men of the people of the city of Pistoia elected and commissioned by the lords Anziani and the Standardbearer

The Elders of Pistoia, "Pistoia: Ordinances for Sanitation in a Time of Mortality," Institute for Advanced Technology in the Humanities, http://jefferson.village.virginia.edu, 2002.

of Justice of the said city concerning the preserving, strengthening and protecting the health of humans from various and diverse pestilences which otherwise can befall the human body. . . .

First. So that no contaminated matter which presently persists in the areas surrounding the city of Pistoia can enter into the bodies of the citizens of Pistoia, these wise men provided and ordered that no citizen of Pistoia or dweller in the district or the county of Pistoia . . . shall in any way dare or presume to go to Pisa or Lucca or to the county or district of either. And that no one can or ought to come from either of them or their districts . . . to the said city of Pistoia or its district or county on penalty of £ 50 . . . And that gatekeeper of the city of Pistoia guarding the gates of the said city shall not permit those coming or returning to the said city of Pistoia from the said cities of Pisa or Lucca, their districts or counties to enter the said gates on penalty of £ 10 . . . It is licit [legal], however, for citizens now living in Pistoia to go to Pisa and Lucca, their districts and counties and then return if they have first obtained a license from the Council of the People. . . .

II. The foresaid wise men provided and ordered that no person whether citizen, inhabitant of the district or county of the city of Pistoia or foreigner shall dare or presume in any way to bring . . . to the city of Pistoia, its district or county, any used cloth, either linen or woolen, for use as clothing for men or women or for bedclothes on penalty of £ 200. . . . Citizens of Pistoia, its district and county returning to the city, district or county will be allowed to bring with them the linen or woolen cloths they are wearing and those for personal use carried in luggage or a small bundle weighing 30 pounds or less. . . . And if any quantity of cloth of the said type or quality has been carried into the said city, county or district, the carrier shall be held to and must remove and export it from the said city, county and district within three days of the adoption of the present ordinance under the foresaid penalty for each carrier or carriers and for each violation.

III. They provided and ordered that the bodies of the dead, after they had died, can not be nor ought to be removed from the place in which they are found unless first such a body has been placed in a wooden casket covered by a lid secured with nails, so that no stench can issue forth from it; nor can it be covered except by a canopy, blanket or drape under a penalty for £ 50 of pennies paid by the heirs of the dead person. . . . And also that likewise such dead bodies of the dead must be carried to the grave only in the said casket under the said penalty as has been said. And so that the foresaid shall be noted by the rectors and officials of the city of Pistoia, present and future rectors of the parishes of the city of Pistoia in whose parish there is any dead person are held to and must themselves announce the death and the district [of the city] in which the dead person lived to the podesta and captain or others of the government of the said city. And they must notify them of the name of the dead person and of the district in which the dead person had lived or pay the said penalty for each contravention. And the podesta and captain to whom such an announcement or notification has been made, immediately are held to and must send one of their officials to the same location to see and inquire if the contents of the present article and other statutes and ordinances concerning funerals are being observed and to punish anyone found culpable according to the said penalty. . . . And the foresaid shall not be enforced nor is it extended to poor and miserable persons who are declared to be poor and miserable according to the form of any statutes or ordinances of the said city.

IV. In order to avoid the foul stench which the bodies of the dead give off they have provided and ordered that any ditch in which a dead body is to be buried must be dug under ground to a depth of 2½ braccia [arm's length] by the measure of the city of Pistoia.

V. They have provided and ordered that no person of whatever condition or status or authority shall dare or presume to return or to carry to the city of Pistoia any dead body in or out of a casket or in any manner on penalty of £ 25 of pennies paid by whoever carries, brings, or orders [a body] to be carried or brought for each occasion. And that the gatekeepers of the said city shall not permit such a body to be sent into the said city on penalty of the foresaid fine by each gatekeeper at the gate through which the said body was sent.

VI. They have provided and ordered that any person who will have come for the burial or to bury any dead person can not and may not be in the presence of the body itself nor with the relatives of such a dead person except for the procession to the church where it will be buried. Nor shall such persons return to the house where the defunct person lived or enter into that house or any other house on the said occasion on penalty of £ 10.

VII. They have provided and ordered that when anyone has died no person should dare or presume to present or to send any gift before or after burial to the former dwelling place of such a dead person or any other place on the said occasion or to attend or to go to a meal in that house or place on the said occasion on penalty of £ 25. . . . Children, carnal brothers and sisters, nieces and nephews of such a dead person and their children, however, shall be excepted [from this provision].

VIII. They have provided and ordered that in order to avoid useless or fruitless expenses no person should dare or presume to dress in new clothing during the period of mourning for any dead person or during the eight days after that, on penalty of £ 25 of pennies for whoever contravenes [this] and for each time. Wives of such dead persons however, shall be exempted; they can be dressed in whatever new clothing they wish without penalty.

IX. They have provided and ordered that no paid mourner . . . shall dare or presume to mourn publicly or privately or to invite other citizens of Pistoia to go to the funeral or to the dead person; nor may anyone engage the foresaid mourner, hornplayer, cryer or drummer.

X. So that the sounds of bells might not depress the infirm nor fear arise in them [the Wise Men] have provided and ordered that the bellringers or custodians in charge of the belltower of the cathedral of Pistoia shall not permit any

bell in the said campanile to be rung for the funeral of the
dead nor shall any person dare or presume to ring any of

New Preventive Measures of Renaissance Italy

*The Black Death prompted new health and sanitation
measures in northern Italy, at the time one of the most industrialized and prosperous regions of Europe. In* Plague
and the Poor in Renaissance Florence, *Ann G. Carmichael
describes the measures taken by the leaders of the Italian
communes (towns) in the fifteenth century to prevent future outbreaks.*

In 1348 Italian communes immediately responded to the
threat of epidemic by enforcing traditional sanitary
laws. When these failed, they enacted extraordinary crisis
measures to minimize social disruption. Finally, they
sought in desperation simply to maintain order through
the disaster. As much as a century later little had changed
in this sequence of responses, despite the frequent recur-
rence of plague.

Then in the mid-fifteenth century, as if by consensus,
Italian legislators decided to isolate plague sufferers by
building or designating a lazaretto (pest house). The em-
phasis on special hospital care shifted from the mere provision of charitable services to isolation of the ill and their
contacts. Once hospital isolation of plague sufferers became routine, lawmakers phrased their concern for plague
control in terms that betrayed their conviction that plague
was a contagious disease. By the end of the fifteenth century health boards were widely considered to be necessary
bureaucracies in overseeing the enforcement of sanitary
law in times of crisis. And, as we have seen, this new leg-
islation had become tinged by the consciousness that
poorer persons were more frequently the victims and the
carriers of plague.

Ann G. Carmichael, *Plague and the Poor in Renaissance Florence.* New York:
Cambridge University Press, 1986.

these bells on the said occasion. . . . At the chapel or parish church of the said dead person or at the friary if the person is to be buried at a church of the friars, they can ring the bell of the chapel, parish church or the church of the friars so long as it is rung only one time and moderately, on the foresaid penalty in the foresaid manner [for each violation].

XI. They have provided and ordered that no one shall dare or presume to gather or cause to gather any persons for the purpose of bringing any widow from the former habitation of a dead person, unless at the time she is being returned from the church or cemetery where such a dead person was buried. [Blood relatives] of such a widow, however, wishing to bring the widow from the house at times other than at the time of burial may send up to four women to accompany the said woman, who is to be brought from the foresaid house of the dead person. . . .

XII. They have provided and ordered that no person should dare or presume to raise or cause to be raised any wailing or clamor over any person or because of any person who has died outside the city, district or county of Pistoia; nor on the said occasion should any persons be brought together in any place except blood relatives and associates of such a dead person, nor on the said occasion should any bell be rung or caused to be wrung, nor announcements be made through the city of Pistoia by mourners, nor on the said occasion should any invitation [to join the mourners] be made on a penalty of £ 25. . . . It must be understood, however, in any written ordinances speaking of the dead and of honoring the burial of the dead that the foresaid shall not have force in the burial of the body of any soldiers of the militia, doctors of laws, judges or physicians whose bodies, because of their dignity, may be honored licitly at burial in a manner pleasing to their heirs.

XIV. They have provided and ordered that butchers and retail vendors of meat, individually and in common, can not, nor ought to hold or maintain near a tavern or other place where they sell meats, or near a shop or beside or behind a shop any stable, pen or any other thing which will give off a putrid smell; nor can they slaughter meat animals nor hang them after slaughter in any stable or other place in which there is any stench on a penalty of £ 10. . . .

XXII. So that stench and putrefaction shall not be harmful to men, henceforth tanning of hides can not and must not be done within the walls of the city of Pistoia on penalty of £ 25. . . .

XXIII. For the observance of each and every provision contained in the present articles and everything in the article speaking of funerals of the dead, of butchers and retail vendors of meats, they provided and ordered that the lord podesta and captain and their officials charged pro tem with the foresaid [duties] shall and must proceed against, investigate, and inquire . . . concerning acts contrary to the foresaid [ordinances], and cause whatever of the foresaid ordained to be reviewed as often as possible, and punish the guilty by the foresaid fines. . . . Also any person may accuse or denounce before either the said podesta or captain any persons acting against the foresaid or any of the foresaid or the content of the said statutes or ordinances. And such denunciations or accusers shall, can and may have one fourth of the fine after it is levied and paid, which fourth part the treasurer pro tem of the treasury of the said city shall be held to and have to pay and give to the said accuser and informer as soon as the fine and penalty have been paid. And sufficient proof shall be offered by one witness worthy of belief, or four persons of good reputation who have learned [of the contravention].

Contending with a New Economy

Anonymous

> The plague brought a radical change in the feudal economy of medieval Europe. As the population decreased, and as serfs and peasants found their labor in high demand, many who had once been tied to the land and to the rural manors of their lords fled their feudal bondage. Some established small estates of their own, while others moved to urban areas, where they freely offered their goods and services to the public.
>
> The following statute, dated June 18, 1349, was passed by the English crown to contend with the changed economy. Free workers were obliged to accept employment, and enjoined not to overcharge for their services. The law required employers not to pay too much in wages and merchants to sell their goods for a reasonable price. In passing these laws, Edward III, the king of England, sought to exercise some control over the rapidly changing laws of supply and demand, which he may have seen as threatening his own authority.

S ince a great part of the population, and especially workers and employees, has now died in this pestilence many people, observing the needs of masters and the shortage of employees, are refusing to work unless they are paid an excessive salary. Others prefer to beg in idleness rather than work for their living. Mindful of the serious inconvenience likely to arise from this shortage, especially of agricultural labourers, we have discussed and considered the matter with

A. Luders et al., *Statutes of the Realm 1101–1713*, vol. I. London, 1810–1828.

our prelates and nobles and other learned men and, with their unanimous advice, we have ordained that every man or woman in our realm of England, whether free or unfree, who is physically fit and below the age of sixty, not living by trade or by exercising a particular craft, and not having private means or land of their own upon which they need to work, and not working for someone else, shall, if offered employment consonant with their status, be obliged to accept the

A Bishop Responds to the Ordinances for Laborers

In response to the ordinance passed by the king, Hamo Hethe, the bishop of Rochester, published the following directive, in which the members of the church are asked to conform to the new law of the land and work for an "appropriate salary."

Recently, the most excellent prince, our illustrious lord the King of England, took action to check the presumptuous excesses of certain artisans and employees. Before the general pestilence of men arose in the kingdom of England and destroyed a great part of the people, such men used to earn their living through various crafts and the work of their hands in a manner very useful to the state, but now that the pestilence has (by God's grace) ceased, although there remain strong and healthy men who are well able to work, yet they obstinately refuse to enter employment or to work unless they receive intolerably high payment for their work or their skill, to the great detriment of the state. With the considered counsel of experienced men and with the benefit of advice from all the other leading men, the king, with their unanimous support, wholesomely ordained appropriate remedies for those matters insofar as they concern lay people, and by his royal writ ordered and caused them to be publicised and their due execution ordered throughout the whole realm of England.

Moreover concerning the stipendiary chaplains and clerks in our said city and diocese who likewise refuse to work employment offered, and they should be paid only the fees, liveries, payments or salaries which were usually paid in the part of the country where they are working in the twentieth year of our reign [1346] or in some other appropriate year five or six years ago. Lords should have first claim on the services of their villeins [serfs] or tenants, although they should retain only as many as they need and no more.

And if any man or woman, being required to enter em-

---

without excessive payment, our lord king ordered us that (insofar as it is our responsibility) we should restrain them from such excess, and compel them to work for an appropriate salary, as is expedient, under pain of suspension and interdict. We have accepted the royal commands, not only because they are supported by reason but also because our office constrains us to exercise our ministry for the public weal, and we therefore order and command you that in every chapter held by you before Michaelmas and in every parish church in our city and diocese you warn each and every stipendiary chaplain and clerk in holy orders celebrating or ministering within our jurisdiction, or ensure that warnings are given to them on your behalf. This is to be done publicly, generally and canonically, so that the admonitions are too forceful to escape notice and nobody can plead ignorance as an excuse. Each one of them is henceforward to be content with the amount of salary or stipend which used to paid before the pestilence for the same type of work in the places where they happen to be employed, and should not dare to demand more. Nor should he presume to withdraw or remove himself from a lord whom he has been serving for an accustomed and appropriate salary, in the hope of obtaining a bigger salary elsewhere, unless he has the special and explicit permission of his lord. These things are to be obeyed under pain of suspension at least, which we will impose on any stipendiary chaplain or clerk contravening or doing anything against the commands set out here.

C. Johnson, ed., *Registrum Hamonis Hethe diocesis Roffensis.* Carlisle, UK: Canterbury and York Society XLVIII, 1948.

ployment in this manner, refuses, and the fact has been proved by two men of legal standing before the sheriff, bailiff or constable of the vill where the incident took place, then let the person be immediately arrested by them or one of them and sent to the nearest gaol, there to remain in close captivity until they offer security that they will accept employment under these conditions.

And no reaper, mower, or other worker or employee of whatever standing who is in the employment of another person shall leave before the end of the agreed period of employment without reasonable cause or permission, under pain of imprisonment, and no one else is to receive or employ him under the same pain of imprisonment.

Fines and Penalties

Moreover, no one should pay or promise wages, liveries [fares], payments or salaries greater than those defined above under pain of paying twice whatever he paid or promised to anyone who feels himself harmed by it. And if no such person is willing to bring a prosecution, then the same to be paid to any member of the public who does so, and let the prosecution be brought in the court of the lord of the place where it happened. And if the lords of vills or manors presume to go against the present ordinance either in person or through their officials, then let them be prosecuted in our county, wapentake [district] or trithing [subcounty] court, or in another of our courts, under penalty of triple the amount paid or promised by them or their officials.

And if it happens that someone, before the present ordinance was made, agreed to enter employment for a larger salary, the employer who made the agreement is not for that reason bound to pay any more than in the past, and should by no means presume to pay more under the abovesaid penalty.

Item, saddlers, skinners, tawyers [tanners], cobblers, tailors, smiths, carpenters, masons, tilers, shipwrights, carters and all other artisans and labourers ought not to receive for their labour and craft more money than they could have expected to receive in the said twentieth year or other appropriate year, in the place where they happen to be working; and if anyone takes more, let him be committed to gaol in the manner set out above.

The Regulation of Prices

Item, butchers, fishmongers, innkeepers, brewers, bakers, poulterers and all other dealers in foodstuffs should be bound to sell the food for a reasonable price, having regard to the price at which such food is sold in the neighbourhood. The price should allow the seller a moderate, but not excessive, profit, taking reasonable account of the distance he has transported the goods. And if a victualler should make a sale contrary to the ordinance, and be convicted for it, then let him pay twice what he has received to the injured party, or, failing him, to the person who has been willing to bring the prosecution. And the mayor and bailiffs of cities, boroughs, market towns and other towns shall have the power to question everyone to discover who has offended against the ordinance, and impose the penalty—which is to be paid to whoever brought the case against the guilty party. And if the mayor and bailiffs neglect to prosecute, and are found guilty before the justices appointed by us, then they should be compelled by the justices to pay damages of triple the value of the goods sold to the injured party or to the other person bringing the prosecution, and also to pay a heavy penalty to us.

And since many sturdy beggars—finding that they can make a living by begging for alms—are refusing to work, and are spending their time instead in idleness and depravity, and sometimes in robberies and other crimes; let no one presume, on pain of imprisonment, to give anything by way of charity or alms to those who are perfectly able to work, or to support them in their idleness, so that they will be forced to work for a living.

We firmly order you that every one of these requirements be proclaimed publicly in the cities, boroughs, market towns, ports and wherever else within your bailliwick you think appropriate, inside franchises as well as outside them.

The Plague Changes English Society

Henry Knighton

The effect of the Black Death on prices and wages was well-chronicled by the English author Henry Knighton, a canon of the abbey of St. Mary of the Meadows in the county of Leicester. Knighton witnessed the plague and writes in great detail of its effect on the people and the cities of England, as well as the effect of a sudden shortage of clergymen to provide the sacraments. In his 1348 chronicle, Knighton reveals that not even the decrees of the king of England could persuade the surviving members of the laboring class from giving up their new advantages in a drastically changed world.

A universal mortality. In this year [1348] and the next there was a general plague upon mankind throughout the world. It began in India, then spread to Tartary [Tartar lands in Russia], and then to the Saracens [of southern Russia and Ukraine], and finally to the Christians and the Jews, so that in the space of a single year, from one Easter to the next, as the report ran in the papal court, some 8,000 legions of people died suddenly in those distant parts, besides Christians.

The king of Tartary proposes to turn Christian. The king of Tartary, seeing the sudden and unparalleled slaughter of his subjects, made his way with a great number of his nobles towards Avignon [in modern France], proposing to turn Christian and be baptized by the pope, as he thought that God's judgement had been visited upon his people for their unbelief. Therefore when he had travelled for twenty days and heard that the plague was as fatal to Christians as to other people he shrewdly turned about, abandoned his journey, and hastened to his own country; but the Christians pursued him and slew some 2,000 of his people.

There died at Avignon in one day, according to a reckoning made before the pope, 1,312, and on another day 400 and more. Of the Dominicans in Provence [a region in southern France] 358 died during Lent [March–April 1348], and of 140 friars at Montpellier only seven survived. At Magdelaine only seven friars remained out of eight score [160] (which was enough). At Marseilles of seven score and ten [150] Minorites, truly, only one remained to tell the tale (and just as well). Of the Carmelites sixty-six perished at Avignon before the citizens knew what was happening, for they were believed to have slain one another. Not one of the Augustinian friars, nor yet their order, survived in Avignon. At the same time the pestilence raged in England, beginning at several places in the autumn, and running through the country to end at the same time the next year. . . .

The Plague in England

Then a lamentable plague travelled by sea to Southampton and on to Bristol, where almost the whole population of the town perished, snatched away, as it were, by sudden death, for there were few who kept their beds for more than two or three days, or even half a day. And thence cruel death spread everywhere with the passage of the sun. There died in Leicester, in the little parish of St Leonard's, more than nineteen score, 400 in the parish of Holy Cross, and in St Margaret's parish 700, and so on in every parish, in great numbers.

The bishop of Lincoln gives chaplains power to absolve. Then the bishop of Lincoln sent word throughout the diocese and gave a general power to all priests, both regular and secular, to hear confessions, and full episcopal authority to absolve, excepting only in matters of debt, in which the debtor should make restitution, if he were able, while he lived, or others should be appointed to do so, with his goods, after his death.

The pope grants a general remission. In the same way the pope granted full remission of all sins to any in danger of death, upon a single occasion, a power which was to last until the following Easter [28 Mar. 1350], and everyone could choose their own confessors at will.

Disease amongst sheep. In the same year there was a great plague amongst sheep everywhere in the realm, so that in one place more than 5,000 died in one pasture, and they so rotted that neither beast not bird would touch them.

A fall in the price of goods. The fear of death caused the price of everything to fall, for there were very few who cared either for wealth or for possessions. A man might have a good horse, which previously would have cost 40*s.*, for half a mark, a heavy, fat ox for 4*s.*, a cow for 12*d.*, a heifer for 6*d.*, a fat sheep for 4*d.*, a ewe for 3*d.*, a lamb for 2*d.*, a great pig for 5*d.*, a stone of wool for 9*d.* And sheep and cattle wandered through the fields and amongst the crops, and there was none to seek them, or round them up, and they perished in out-of-the-way places amongst the furrows and under hedges, for want of a keeper, in numbers beyond reckoning throughout the land, for there was such a shortage of hands and servants that no one knew what ought to be done.

For there was no memory of so unsparing and savage a plague since the days of Vortigern, king of the Britons, in whose time, as Bede [a saint and chronicler of the seventh and eighth centuries] records in his history of the English, there were not enough left alive to bury the dead. In the following autumn no one could hire a mower for less than 8*d.* with his keep, or a reaper for less than 12*d.* with his keep. So many crops rotted in the fields for want of harvesting, but in the year of the plague, as has been said already, in another connection, there was such an abundance of grain that almost no one cared for it.

The Scots mock the English over the plague. The Scots, hearing of the cruel plague amongst the English, attributed it to the avenging hand of God, and took it up as an oath, as a common report came to English ears, and when they wished to swear they would say 'By the filthy death of England' (or in English: 'Be the foul deth of Engelond'). And thus the Scots, believing God's dreadful judgement to have descended upon the English, gathered in the forest of Selkirk ready to over run the whole kingdom of England. And a fierce pestilence arose, and blew a sudden and monstrous death upon the Scots, and some 5,000 of them died in a short time, and the rest of them, some fit and some enfeebled, prepared to make their way home, but the English pursued them and fell upon them, and slew a great many of them.

Master Thomas Bradwardine was consecrated archbishop of Canterbury by the pope, and when he returned to England he came to London, and within two days he was dead. He was celebrated beyond all the scholars of Christendom, in theology pre-eminently, but also in all other liberal learning.

A Rise in Wages

At that time there was such a shortage of priests everywhere that many churches were bereft of the divine office: of masses, matins, and vespers, of sacraments and observances. A man could scarcely retain a chaplain to serve a church for less than £10, or perhaps 10 marks, and where one might have had a chaplain for four or five marks, or two marks and his keep, with such numbers of priests as there were about before the plague, now in those times there was almost no one willing to take a vicarage for £20, or perhaps 20 marks. But within a short time there came into holy orders a great multitude of those whose wives had died in the plague, many of them illiterate, the merest laymen, who if they were able to read at all were unable to understand what they read.

Ox hides fell to a wretched price, namely 12*d.*, and yet a pair of gloves would cost 10*d.*, 12*d.*, or 14*d.*, and a pair of breeches 3*s.* or 4*s.* In the mean time the king sent word into every shire that mowers and other workmen should take no more than they had before, under the penalties laid down in the order, and thereupon made a statute. Nevertheless the workmen were so puffed up and contrary-minded that they did not heed the king's decree, and if anyone wanted to hire them he had to pay what they asked: either his fruit and crops rotted, or he had to give in to the workmen's arrogant and greedy demands.

When it came to the king's notice that they had not obeyed his order, and had given their employees higher wages, he inflicted heavy fines upon abbots and priors, and upon greater and lesser knights, and upon the others, great

The Plague Corrects Overpopulation

One important scientific theory states that the Black Death and other such epidemics are nature's way of correcting the problem of overpopulation. Charles T. Gregg, in Plague! The Shocking Story of a Dread Disease in America Today, *makes the case that a similar corrective may occur in the modern world.*

No one can say with certainty why the pandemic ceased when it did, but it is clear that when the Black Death arrived, Europe offered it fertile soil. By the early fourteenth century, the population of the Continent had risen rapidly, far more rapidly than the food supply. Soon bad harvests reduced the poor to eating dogs and cats, perhaps even their own children. Even before the Black Death, Europe was in the clammy grip of a vast depression, and the population had declined slightly. But starvation is a slow and clumsy corrective for overpopulation. Plague is fast and efficient. The Black Death slaughtered one of every four Europeans; subsequent epidemics raised the toll to one in three. The surplus population, for which there was little employment and less food, was efficiently consumed by plague. Unless gentler correctives to overpopulation are effective in time, the lesson of the Black Death may be repeated in this century.

Charles T. Gregg, *Plague! The Shocking Story of a Dread Disease in America Today.* New York: Charles Scribner's Sons, 1978.

and small, of the land: from some 100s., from some 20s., and from each according to what he could pay. And he took 20s from every ploughland [fertile field] in the kingdom, and received not less than a fifteenth would yield [in taxes].

Then the king caused many labourers to be arrested, and put them in prison. Many ran away, and took to the woods and forests for a time, but those who were caught were grievously fined. And most were sworn that they would not take more than the old established daily rate, and so were freed from prison. And artisans in the boroughs and townships were treated in the same way. . . .

After the plague many buildings, both large and small, in all the cities, boroughs, and townships, decayed and were utterly razed to the ground for want of occupants, and similarly many villages and hamlets were deserted with not a house left in them, for all who had lived there were dead, and it is likely that many of those villages will never he inhabited again.

In the following winter there was such a want of hands, for every kind of work, that people believed that the like shortage had never been known at any time in the past, for cattle and such livestock as a man might have wandered about without a keeper, and there was no one to look after people's possessions. And thus the necessities of life became so dear, that what in previous times was worth 1d. now cost 4d. or 5d.

Lords remit their tenants' rent. Whereupon both the magnates of the realm, and also lesser lords who had tenants, remitted the payment of rents lest their tenants should quit for want of labour, and the high cost of living: some half the rent, some more or less, some for two years, some for three, some for one, according to what they could agree.

Similarly those who had tenants with day-work throughout the year, such as bondmen, had to relax and remit such works, and either give them up altogether, or manage them in a looser way, at a low rent, lest their tenements should fall into utter and irredeemable decay, and the land everywhere lie wholly unworked. And foodstuffs and necessities of all kinds became vastly dear.

The King Prevents Travel

A general absolution. In the year of grace 1349 a general indulgence [absolution of sins] began at Rome, and many prepared to travel there, but the king forbade their journey because of the [Hundred Years'] war with France. Whereupon the pope sent ambassadors to the king, chiefly to procure the right to travel. And they asked firstly, that the king should not impede the holy travel of those who wished to visit the sacred places of the Apostles; and also that he should grant a truce lest the earl of Lancaster should ride in Aquitaine to the danger of those seeking to visit the holy places. And similarly that the king should neither prevent, nor allow others to prevent, those promoted by papal bull receiving the benefices bestowed upon them.

And to the first article the king answered that he was engaged in a war, and needed supplies, and that while the war lasted he had to look to the treasure of his realm lest it should, to the prejudice of himself and his subjects, be taken out of the realm. Thereupon the king had it proclaimed that all Englishmen, in Rome and elsewhere overseas, should return as speedily as they could, upon pain of forfeiting their persons and all their possessions.

To the second article, touching provisors, it was answered that the king would readily accept such clergy provided that they were of good repute, and worthy of provision, but otherwise not. To the third article, about a truce, it was answered that the king of France often during such truces would ride treacherously upon the king of England's lands, to the destruction of the people and contrary to the provisions of the truce. And with that answer the pope's envoys went home.

Chapter 5

The Plague Year in London

Chapter Preface

The bubonic plague remained a frequent visitor to the cities of Europe for centuries after the Black Death of the fourteenth century. Most of the time the disease remained dormant, but about once in a generation, another European city would experience the disease. In 1665 a plague epidemic struck London, then the economic and commercial capital of the British Isles and Europe. The plague had appeared in Holland two years earlier, yet despite a total ban on trade with the Low Countries by the English king Charles II, the disease made its way across the English Channel.

Science had made many important advances since the time of the Black Death, but no one yet guessed at the existence of the plague bacillus, now known as *Yersinia pestis*, nor did anyone have any idea how to prevent or treat the disease. The plague was just as terrifying and just as fatal in the seventeenth century as it had been in the fourteenth. By July 1665 more than a thousand people were dying in London every week, and the toll rose to more than six thousand a week by August. Plague victims were shut up in their houses with their families, with a guard posted outside to prevent anyone from escaping or entering the house. Suspected of carrying the disease, stray cats and dogs were killed, giving the plague-carrying rats a respite from their natural enemies.

The plague finally subsided in the winter of 1665, yet London was not yet free of disaster. In September 1666 the Great Fire would strike, burning four out of five London homes to the ground. The fire, at least, was well understood as the fault of a careless employee in a bakery. The plague would not be understood for more than two centuries afterward.

A Literary Account of the Plague

Daniel Defoe

The English author Daniel Defoe, who was four years old at the time of the London plague outbreak of 1665, documented the plague's effects in a book originally titled *A Journal of the Plague Year: Being Observations or Memorials of the Most Remarkable Occurrences, As Well Public as Private, Which Happened in London During the Last Great Visitation in 1665.* For the popularity of his work, Defoe was counting on a renewed public fear of the plague, which had recently reappeared in the French port of Marseille.

For this work Defoe drew on the reminiscences of his own family, as well as books on the 1665 outbreak which he kept in his own library. He creates a first-person narrator to realistically describe the events taking place in the London streets and neighborhoods where the plague was raging. As in his other works, Defoe uses surface events to probe human behavior and to draw important moral lessons for his readers. His semifictional account, first published in 1722, has become a literary classic and one of the most famous examples of "plague literature," which probes the social disruptions caused by deadly pestilences such as the Black Death.

I went all the first part of the time freely about the streets, though not so freely as to run myself into apparent danger, except when they dug the great pit in the churchyard of our parish of Aldgate. A terrible pit it was, and I could not

Daniel Defoe, *A Journal of the Plague Year*. London: J.M. Dent and Sons, 1908.

resist my curiosity to go and see it. As near as I may judge, it was about forty feet in length, and about fifteen or sixteen feet broad, and at the time I first looked at it, about nine feet deep; but it was said they dug it near twenty feet deep afterwards in one part of it, till they could go no deeper for the water; for they had, it seems, dug several large pits before this. For though the plague was long a-coming to our parish, yet, when it did come, there was no parish in or about London where it raged with such violence as in the two parishes of Aldgate and Whitechapel.

I say they had dug several pits in another ground, when the distemper [plague] began to spread in our parish, and especially when the dead-carts began to go about, which was not, in our parish, till the beginning of August. Into these pits they had put perhaps fifty or sixty bodies each; then they made larger holes, wherein they buried all that the cart brought in a week, which, by the middle to the end of August, came to from 200 to 400 a week; and they could not well dig them larger, because of the order of the magistrates confining them to leave no bodies within six feet of the surface; and the water coming on at about seventeen or eighteen feet, they could not well, I say, put more in one pit. But now, at the beginning of September, the plague raging in a dreadful manner, and the number of burials in our parish increasing to more than was ever buried in any parish about London of no larger extent, they ordered this dreadful gulf to be dug, for such it was rather than a pit.

They had supposed this pit would have supplied them for a month or more when they dug it, and some blamed the churchwardens for suffering such a frightful thing, telling them they were making preparations to bury the whole parish, and the like; but time made it appear the churchwardens knew the condition of the parish better than they did, for the pit being finished the 4th of September, I think, they began to bury in it the 6th, and by the 20th, which was just two weeks, they had thrown into it 1114 bodies, when they were obliged to fill it up, the bodies being then come to lie within six feet of the surface. I doubt not but there may be some ancient persons alive in the parish who can justify the fact of this, and are able to show even in what place of the churchyard the pit lay better than I can. The mark of it also was many years to be seen in the churchyard on the surface, lying in length parallel with the passage which goes by the west wall of the churchyard out of Houndsditch, and turns east again into Whitechapel, coming out near the Three Nuns' Inn.

Visiting the Burial Pit

It was about the 10th of September that my curiosity led, or rather drove, me to go and see this pit again, when there had been near 400 people buried in it; and I was not content to see it in the day-time, as I had done before, for then there would have been nothing to have been seen but the loose earth; for all the bodies that were thrown in were immediately covered with earth by those they called the buriers, which at other times were called bearers; but I resolved to go in the night and see some of them thrown in.

There was a strict order to prevent people coming to those pits, and that was only to prevent infection. But after some time that order was more necessary, for people that were infected and near their end, and delirious also, would run to those pits, wrapt in blankets or rugs, and throw themselves in, and, as they said, bury themselves. I cannot say that the officers suffered any willingly to lie there; but I have heard that in a great pit in Finsbury, in the parish of Cripplegate, it lying open then to the fields, for it was not then walled about, [some] came and threw themselves in, and expired there, before they threw any earth upon them; and that when they came to bury others, and found them there, they were quite dead, though not cold.

This may serve a little to describe the dreadful condition of that day, though it is impossible to say anything that is able to give a true idea of it to those who did not see it, other than this, that it was indeed very, very, very dreadful, and such as no tongue can express.

I got admittance into the churchyard by being acquainted

with the sexton who attended, who, though he did not refuse me at all, yet earnestly persuaded me not to go, telling me very seriously, for he was a good, religious, and sensible man, that it was indeed their business and duty to venture, and to run all hazards, and that in it they might hope to be preserved; but that I had no apparent call to it but my own curiosity, which, he said, he believed I would not pretend was sufficient to justify my running that hazard. I told him I had been pressed in my mind to go, and that perhaps it might be an instructing sight, that might not be without its uses. "Nay," says the good man, "if you will venture upon that score, name of God go in; for, depend upon it, t'will be a sermon to you, it may be, the best that ever you heard in your life. 'Tis a speaking sight," says he, "and has a voice with it, and a loud one, to call us all to repentance;" and with that he opened the door and said, "Go, if you will."

His discourse had shocked my resolution a little, and I stood wavering for a good while, but just at that interval I saw two links come over from the end of the Minories, and heard the bellman, and then appeared a dead-cart, as they called it, coming over the streets; so I could no longer resist my desire of seeing it, and went in. There was nobody, as I could perceive at first, in the churchyard, or going into it, but the buriers and the fellow that drove the cart, or rather led the horse and cart; but when they came up to the pit they saw a man go to and again, muffled up in a brown cloak, and making motions with his hands under his cloak, as if he was in a great agony, and the buriers immediately gathered about him, supposing he was one of those poor delirious or desperate creatures that used to pretend, as I have said, to bury themselves. He said nothing as he walked about, but two or three times groaned very deeply and loud, and sighed as he would break his heart.

Mournful Scenes

When the buriers came up to him they soon found he was neither a person infected and desperate, as I have observed above, or a person distempered in mind, but one oppressed with a dreadful weight of grief indeed, having his wife and several of his children all in the cart that was just come in with him, and he followed in an agony and excess of sorrow. He mourned heartily, as it was easy to see, but with a kind of masculine grief that could not give itself vent by tears; and calmly defying the buriers to let him alone, said he would only see the bodies thrown in and go away, so they left importuning him. But no sooner was the cart turned round and the bodies shot into the pit promiscuously, which was a surprise to him, for he at least expected they would have been decently laid in, though indeed he was afterwards convinced that was impracticable; I say, no sooner did he see the sight but he cried out aloud, unable to contain himself. I could not hear what he said, but he went backward two or three steps and fell down in a swoon. The buriers ran to him and took him up, and in a little while he came to himself, and they led him away to the Pie Tavern over against the end of Houndsditch, where, it seems, the man was known, and where they took care of him. He looked into the pit again as he went away, but the buriers had covered the bodies so immediately with throwing in earth, that though there was light enough, for there were lanterns, and candles in them, placed all night round the sides of the pit, upon heaps of earth, seven or eight, or perhaps more, yet nothing could be seen.

This was a mournful scene indeed, and affected me almost as much as the rest; but the other was awful and full of terror. The cart had in it sixteen or seventeen bodies; some were wrapt up in linen sheets, some in rags, some little other than naked, or so loose that what covering they had fell from them in the shooting out of the cart, and they fell quite naked among the rest; but the matter was not much to them, or the indecency much to any one else, seeing they were all dead, and were to be huddled together into the common grave of mankind, as we may call it, for here was no difference made, but poor and rich went together; there was no other way of burials, neither was it possible there should, for coffins were not to be had for the prodigious numbers that fell in such a calamity as this.

It was reported by way of scandal upon the buriers, that if any corpse was delivered to them decently wound up, as we called it then, in a winding-sheet tied over the head and feet, which some did, and which was generally of good linen; I say, it was reported that the buriers were so wicked as to strip them in the cart and carry them quite naked to the ground. But as I cannot easily credit anything so vile among Christians, and at a time so filled with terrors as that was, I can only relate it and leave it undetermined.

Innumerable stories also went about of the cruel behaviours and practices of nurses who tended the sick, and of their hastening on the fate of those they tended in their sickness. But I shall say more of this in its place.

I was indeed shocked with this sight; it almost overwhelmed me, and I went away with my heart most afflicted, and full of the afflicting thoughts, such as I cannot describe. Just at my going out of the church, and turning up the street towards my own house, I saw another cart with links, and a bellman going before, coming out of Harrow Alley in the Butcher Row, on the other side of the way, and being, as I perceived, very full of dead bodies, it went directly over the street also toward the church. I stood a while, but I had no stomach to go back again to see the same dismal scene over again, so I went directly home, where I could not but consider with thankfulness the risk I had run, believing I had gotten no injury, as indeed I had not.

Here the poor unhappy gentleman's grief came into my head again, and indeed I could not but shed tears in the reflection upon it, perhaps more than he did himself; but his case lay so heavy upon my mind that I could not prevail with myself, but that I must go out again into the street, and go to the Pie Tavern, resolving to inquire what became of him.

Ruffians Mock the Plague

It was by this time one o'clock in the morning, and yet the poor gentleman was there. The truth was, the people of the house, knowing him, had entertained him, and kept him there all the night, notwithstanding the danger of being infected by him, though it appeared the man was perfectly sound himself.

It is with regret that I take notice of this tavern. The people were civil, mannerly, and an obliging sort of folks enough, and had till this time kept their house open and their trade going on, though not so very publicly as formerly; but there was a dreadful set of fellows that used their house, and who, in the middle of all this horror, met there every night, behaved with all the revelling and roaring extravagances as is usual for such people to do at other times, and, indeed, to such an offensive degree that the very master and mistress of the house grew first ashamed and then terrified at them.

They sat generally in a room next the street, and as they always kept late hours, so when the dead-cart came across the street-end to go into Houndsditch, which was in view of the tavern windows, they would frequently open the windows as soon as they heard the bell and look out at them; and as they might often hear sad lamentations of people in the streets or at their windows as the carts went along, they would make their impudent mocks and jeers at them, especially if they heard the poor people call upon God to have mercy upon them, as many would do at those times in their ordinary passing along the streets.

These gentlemen, being something disturbed with the clutter of bringing the poor gentleman into the house, as above, were first angry and very high with the master of the house for suffering such a fellow, as they called him, to be brought out of the grave into their house; but being answered that the man was a neighbour, and that he was sound, but overwhelmed with the calamity of his family, and the like, they turned their anger into ridiculing the man and his sorrow for his wife and children, taunted him with want of courage to leap into the great pit and go to heaven, as they jeeringly expressed it, along with them, adding some very profane and even blasphemous expressions.

They were at this vile work when I came back to the house, and, as far as I could see, though the man sat still, mute and disconsolate, and their affronts could not divert his sorrow, yet he was both grieved and offended at their discourse. Upon this I gently reproved them, being well enough acquainted with their characters, and not unknown in person to two of them.

They immediately fell upon me with ill language and oaths, asked me what I did out of my grave at such a time when so many honester men were carried into the churchyard, and why I was not at home saying my prayers against the dead-cart came for me, and the like.

I was indeed astonished at the impudence of the men, though not at all discomposed at their treatment of me. However, I kept my temper. I told them that though I defied them or any man in the world to tax me with any dishonesty, yet I acknowledged that in this terrible judgment of God many better than I were swept away and carried to their grave. But to answer their question directly, the case was, that I was mercifully preserved by that great God whose name they had blasphemed and taken in vain by cursing and swearing in a dreadful manner, and that I believed I was preserved in particular, among other ends of His goodness, that I might reprove them for their audacious boldness in behaving in such a manner and in such an awful time as this was, especially for their jeering and mocking at an honest gentleman and a neighbour (for some of them knew him), who, they saw, was overwhelmed with sorrow for the breaches which it had pleased God to make upon his family.

Jesting at the Name of God

I cannot call exactly to mind the hellish, abominable raillery which was the return they made to that talk of mine, being provoked, it seems, that I was not at all afraid to be free with them; nor, if I could remember, would I fill my account with any of the words, the horrid oaths, curses, and vile expressions, such as, at that time of the day, even the worst and ordinariest people in the street would not use; for, except such hardened creatures as these, the most wicked wretches that could be found had at that time some terror upon their minds of the hand of that Power which could thus in a moment destroy them.

But that which was the worst in all their devilish language was, that they were not afraid to blaspheme God and talk atheistically, making a jest of my calling the plague the hand of God; mocking, and even laughing, at the word judgment, as if the providence of God had no concern in the inflicting such a desolating stroke, and that the people calling upon God as they saw the carts carrying away the dead bodies was all enthusiastic, absurd, and impertinent.

I made them some reply, such as I thought proper, but which I found was so far from putting a check to their horrid way of speaking that it made them rail the more, so that I confess it filled me with horror and a kind of rage, and I came away, as I told them, lest the hand of that Judgment which had visited the whole city should glorify His vengeance upon them, and all that were near them.

They received all reproof with the utmost contempt, and made the greatest mockery that was possible for them to do at me, giving me all the opprobrious, insolent scoffs that they could think of for preaching to them, as they called it, which indeed grieved me, rather than angered me; and I went away, blessing God, however, in my mind that I had not spared them, though they had insulted me so much.

They continued this wretched course three or four days after this, continually mocking and jeering at all that showed themselves religious or serious, or that were any way touched with the sense of the terrible judgment of God upon us; and I was informed they flouted in the same manner at the good people who, notwithstanding the contagion, met at the church, fasted, and prayed to God to remove His hand from them.

I say, they continued this dreadful course three or four days—I think it was no more—when one of them, particularly he who asked the poor gentleman what he did out of his grave, was struck from Heaven with the plague, and died in a most deplorable manner; and, in a word, they were every one of them carried into the great pit which I have mentioned above, before it was quite filled up, which was not above a fortnight or thereabout.

These men were guilty of many extravagances, such as one would think human nature should have trembled at the thoughts of at such a time of general terror as was then upon us, and particularly scoffing and mocking at everything which they happened to see that was religious among the people, especially at their thronging zealously to the place of public worship to implore mercy from Heaven in such a time of distress; and this tavern where they held their club being within view of the church-door, they had the more particular occasion for their atheistical profane mirth. . . .

Shutting Up the Houses

But I must go back here to the particular incidents which occur to my thoughts of the time of the visitation, and particularly to the time of their shutting up houses, in the first part of their sickness; for before the sickness was come to its height people had more room to make their observations than they had afterward; but when it was in the extremity there was no such thing as communication with one another, as before.

During the shutting up of houses, as I have said, some violence was offered to the watchmen. . . .

This made the watchmen be the less regarded, and perhaps occasioned the greater violence to be used against them. I mention it on this score to observe that the setting watchmen thus to keep the people in was, first of all, not effectual, but that the people broke out, whether by force or by stratagem, even almost as often as they pleased; and, second, that those that did thus break out were generally people infected, who, in their desperation, running about from one place to another, valued not whom they injured, and which perhaps, as I have said, might give birth to report that it was natural to the infected people to desire to infect others, which report was really false.

And I know it so well, and in so many several cases, that I could give several relations of good, pious, and religious people who, when they have had the distemper, have been so far from being forward to infect others that they have forbid their own family to come near them, in hopes of their being preserved, and have even died without seeing their nearest relations lest they should be instrumental to give them the distemper, and infect or endanger them. If, then, there were cases wherein the infected people were careless of the injury they did to others, this was certainly one of them, if not the chief, namely, when people who had the distemper had broken out from houses which were so shut up, and having been driven to extremities for provision or for entertainment, had endeavoured to conceal their condition, and have been thereby instrumental involuntarily to infect others who have been ignorant and unwary.

This is one of the reasons why I believed then, and do believe still, that the shutting up houses thus by force, and restraining, or rather imprisoning, people in their own houses, as I said above, was of little or no service in the whole. Nay, I am of opinion it was rather hurtful, having forced those desperate people to wander abroad with the plague upon them, who would otherwise have died quietly in their beds.

I remember one citizen who, having thus broken out of his house in Aldersgate Street or thereabout, went along the road to Islington; he attempted to have gone in at the Angel Inn, and after that the White Horse, two inns known still by the same signs, but was refused; after which he came to the Pied Bull, an inn also still continuing the same sign. He asked them for lodging for one night only, pretending to be going into Lincolnshire, and assuring them of his being very sound and free from the infection, which also at that time had not reached much that way.

They told him they had no lodging that they could spare but one bed up in the garret, and that they could spare that bed for one night, some drovers being expected the next day with cattle; so, if he would accept of that lodging, he might have it, which he did. So a servant was sent up with a candle with him to show him the room. He was very well dressed, and looked like a person not used to lie in a garret; and when he came to the room he fetched a deep sigh, and said to the servant, "I have seldom lain in such a lodging as this." However, the servant assuring him again that they had no better, "Well," says he, "I must make shift; this is a dreadful time; but it is but for one night." So he sat down upon the bedside, and bade the maid, I think it was, fetch him up a pint of warm ale. Accordingly the servant went for the ale, but some hurry in the house, which perhaps employed her other ways, put it out of her head, and she went up no more to him.

The next morning, seeing no appearance of the gentleman, somebody in the house asked the servant that had showed him upstairs what was become of him. She started. "Alas!" says she, "I never thought more of him. He bade me carry him some warm ale, but I forgot." Upon which, not the maid, but some other person was sent up to see after him, who, coming into the room, found him stark dead and almost cold, stretched out across the bed. His clothes were pulled off, his jaw fallen, his eyes open in a most frightful posture, the rug of the bed being grasped hard in one of his hands, so that it was plain he died soon after the maid left him; and 'tis probable, had she gone up with the ale, she had found him dead in a few minutes after he sat down upon the bed. The alarm was great in the house, as any one may suppose, they having been free from the distemper till that disaster, which, bringing the infection to the house, spread it immediately to other houses round about it. I do not remember how many died in the house itself, but I think the maid-servant who went up first with him fell presently ill by the fright, and several others; for, whereas there died but two in Islington of the plague the week before, there died seventeen the week after, whereof fourteen were of the plague. This was in the week from the 11th of July to the 18th. . . .

Carelessness Spreads the Plague

I must here take further notice that nothing was more fatal to the inhabitants of this city than the supine negligence of the people themselves, who, during the long notice or warning they had of the visitation, made no provision for it, by laying in store of provisions, or of other necessaries, by which they might have lived retired, and within their own houses, as I have observed others did, and who were in a great measure preserved by that caution; nor were they, after they were a little hardened to it, so shy of conversing with one another, when actually infected, as they were at first, no, though they knew it.

I acknowledge I was one of those thoughtless ones that had made so little provision that my servants were obliged to go out of doors to buy every trifle by penny and half-penny, just as before it began, even till my experience showing me the folly, I began to be wiser so late that I had scarce time to store myself sufficient for our common subsistence for a month.

I had in family only an ancient woman that managed the house, a maid-servant, two apprentices, and myself; and the plague beginning to increase about us, I had many sad thoughts about what course I should take, and how I should act. The many dismal objects, which happened everywhere as I went about the streets, had filled my mind with a great deal of horror, for fear of the distemper, which was, indeed, very horrible in itself, and in some more than in others. The swellings, which were generally in the neck or groin, when they grew hard and would not break, grew so painful that it was equal to the most exquisite torture; and some, not able to bear the torment, threw themselves out at windows or shot themselves, or otherwise made themselves away, and I saw several dismal objects of that kind. Others, unable to contain themselves, vented their pain by incessant roarings, and such loud and lamentable cries were to be heard as we walked along the streets that would pierce the very heart to think of, especially when it was to be considered that the same dreadful scourge might be expected every moment to seize upon ourselves.

Daily Life and the Plague

Samuel Pepys

Samuel Pepys, clerk of the Acts of the Navy Board, held an influential position in the royal bureaucracy of seventeenth-century England. He was well known to the king and the court of England, but his literary fame rests on his lengthy diary and his ability to take down the minute details of his everyday life in sometimes exhausting detail. By reading Pepys' diary, the modern student of historical London can take a vivid tour of life as it was lived more than three centuries ago and grow closely acquainted with Pepys' opinions, emotions, and outlook on life.

Pepys, who was born in 1633, experienced firsthand the London plague of 1665. In the following diary extracts, he describes what he saw, his own moody cast of mind at the thought of his own mortality, and the general fear and chaos that took place as the disease gripped the city.

[June] 10th. In the evening home to supper; and there, to my great trouble, hear that the plague is come into the City (though it hath these three or four weeks since its beginning been wholly out of the City); but where should it begin but in my good friend and neighbour's, Dr. Burnett, in Fanchurch Street: which in both points troubles me mightily. To the office to finish my letters and then home to bed, being troubled at the sicknesse, and my head filled also with other business enough, and particularly how to put my

Samuel Pepys, *Passages from the Diary of Samuel Pepys*, edited by Richard Le Gallienne. New York: Carlton House.

things and estate in order, in case it should please God to call me away, which God dispose of to his glory.

11th (Lord's day). . . . I out of doors a little, to shew, forsooth, my new suit, and back again, and in going I saw poor Dr. Burnett's door shut; but he hath, I hear, gained great goodwill among his neighbours; for he discovered it himself first, and caused himself to be shut up of his own accord: which was very handsome.

15th. The towne grows very sickly, and people to be afeard of it; there dying this last week of the plague 112, from 43 the week before, whereof but [one] in Fanchurchstreete, and one in Broad-streete, by the Treasurer's office.

16th. I to White Hall, where the Court is full of the Duke and his courtiers returned from sea. All fat and lusty, and ruddy by being in the sun.

17th. It struck me very deep this afternoon going with a hackney coach from my Lord Treasurer's down Holborne, the coachman I found to drive easily and easily, at last stood still, and come down hardly able to stand, and told me that he was suddenly struck very sicke, and almost blind, he could not see; so I [a]'light and went into another coach, with a sad heart for the poor man and trouble for myself, lest he should have been struck with the plague, being at the end of the towne that I took him up; but God have mercy upon us all!

20th. This day I informed myself that there died four or five at Westminster of the plague in one alley in several house upon Sunday last, Bell Alley, over against the Palacegate; yet people do think that the number will be fewer in the towne than it was the last weeke.

21st. So homewards and to the Cross Keys at Cripplegate, where I find all the towne almost going out of the towne, the coaches and waggons being all full of people going into the country. Here I had some of the company of the tapster's wife a while, and so home to my office, and then home to supper and to bed.

23rd. So home by hackney coach, which is become a very dangerous passage now-a-days, the sickness increasing mightily, and to bed.

26th. The plague encreases mightily, I this day seeing a house, at a bitt-maker's over against St. Clement's Church, in the open street, shut up; which is a sad sight.

29th. Up and by water to White Hall, where the Court full of waggons and people ready to go out of towne. To the Harp and Ball, and there drank and talked with Mary, she telling me in discourse that she lived lately at my neighbour's, Mr. Knightly, which made me forbear further discourse. This end of the towne every day grows very bad of the plague. The Mortality Bill is come to 267; which is about ninety more than the last: and of these but four in the City, which is a great blessing to us.

30th. Thus this book of two years ends. Myself and family in good health, consisting of myself and wife, Mercer, her woman, Mary, Alice, and Susan our maids, and Tom my boy. In a sickly time of the plague growing on. Having upon my hands the troublesome care of the Treasury of Tangier, with great sums drawn upon me, and nothing to pay them with: also the business of the office great. Consideration of removing my wife to Woolwich; she lately busy in learning to paint, with great pleasure and successe. All other things well; especially a new interest I am making, by a match in hand between the eldest son of Sir G. Carteret, and my Lady Jeminah Montagu.

July 1st, 1665. To Westminster, where I hear the sicknesse encreases greatly. Sad at the newes that seven or eight houses in Bazing Hall street, are shut up of the plague.

3rd. Resolving from this night forwards to close all my letters, if possible, and end all my business at the office by daylight, and I shall go near to do it and put all my affairs in the world in good order, the season growing so sickly, that it is much to be feared how a man can escape having a share with others in it, for which the good Lord God bless me, or to be fitted to receive it. So after supper to bed, and mightily troubled in my sleep all night with dreams of Jacke Cole, my old schoolfellow, lately dead, who was born at the same time with me, and we reckoned our fortunes pretty equal. God fit me for his condition!

7th. Up, and having set my neighbour, Mr. Hudson, wine coopers, at work drawing out a tirce [42 gallons] of wine for the sending of some of it to my wife, I abroad, only taking notice to what a condition it hath pleased God to bring me that at this time I have two tierces of Claret [French Bordeaux wine], two quarter casks of Canary, and a smaller vessel of Sack; a vessel of Tent, another of Malaga, and another of white wine, all in my wine cellar together; which, I believe, none of my friends of my name now alive ever had of his owne at one time.

10th. Up, and with great pleasure looking over a nest of puppies of Mr. Sheldon's, with which my wife is most extraordinary pleased, and one of them is promised her.

12th. After doing what business I could in the morning, it being a solemn fast-day for the plague growing upon us, I took boat and down to Deptford, where I stood with great pleasure an houre or two by my Lady Sandwich's bedside, talking to her (she lying prettily in bed).

18th. I was much troubled this day to hear at Westminster how the officers do bury the dead in the open Tuttle-fields, pretending want of room elsewhere; whereas the New Chappell church-yard was walled-in at the publick charge in the last plague-time, merely for want of room and now none, but such as are able to pay dear for it, can be buried there.

21st. So home and late at my chamber, setting some papers in order; the plague growing very raging, and my apprehensions of it great. So very late to bed.

26th. Up, and after doing a little business, down to Deptford with Sir W. Batten, and there left him, and I to Greenwich to the Park, where I hear the King and Duke are come by water this morn from Hampton Court. They asked me several questions. The King mightily pleased with his new buildings there. Down to Woolwich (and there I just saw and kissed my wife, and saw some of her painting, which is very curious; and away again to the King) and back again with him in the barge, hearing him and the Duke talk, and seeing and observing their manner of discourse. And God forgive me! though I admire them with all the duty possible, yet the more a man considers and observes them, the less he finds of difference between them and other men, though (blessed be God!) they are both princes of great nobleness and spirits. Duke of Monmouth is the most skittish leaping gallant that ever I saw, always in action, vaulting or leaping, or clambering. The sicknesse is got into our parish this week, and is got, indeed, every where; so that I begin to think of setting things in order, which I pray God enable me to put both as to soul and body.

28th. Up betimes [early], and down to Deptford, where, after a little discourse with Sir G. Carteret. Set out with my Lady all alone with her with six horses to Dagenhams; going by water to the Ferry. And a pleasant going, and good discourse; and when there, very merry, and the young couple now well acquainted. But, Lord! to see in what fear all the people here do live would make one mad, they are afeard of us that come to them, insomuch that I am troubled at it, and wish myself away. But some cause they have; for the chaplin, with whom but a week or two ago we were here mighty high disputing, is since fallen into a fever and dead, being gone hence to a friend's a good way off. A sober and a healthful man. These considerations make us all hasten the marriage, and resolve it upon Monday next, which is three days before we intended it. Mighty merry all of us, and in the evening with full content took coach again and home by daylight with great pleasure, and thence I down to Woolwich, where find my wife well, and after drinking and talking a little we to bed.

30th (Lord's day). It was a sad noise to hear our bell to toll and ring so often to-day, either for deaths or burnals; I think five or six times. At night weary with my day's work, but full of joy at my having done it, I to bed, being to rise betimes to-morrow to go to the wedding at Dagenhams. . . .

10th. By and by to the office, where we sat all the morning; in great trouble to see the Bill this week rise so high, to above 4,000 in all, and of them above 3,000 of the plague. And an odd story of Alderman Bence's stumbling at night over a dead corps in the street, and going home and telling his wife, she at the fright, being with child, fell sicke and died of the plague. Thence to the office and, after writing letters, home, to draw over anew my will, which I had bound myself by oath to dispatch by to-morrow night; the town growing so unhealthy, that a man cannot depend upon living two days to an end. . . .

12th. The people die so, that now it seems they are fain to carry the dead to be buried by day-light, the nights not sufficing to do it in. And my Lord Mayor commands people to be within at nine at night all, as they say, that the sick may have liberty to go abroad for ayre.

14th. This night I did present my wife with the dyamond ring, awhile since given me by Mr. Dicke Vines's brother, for helping him to be a purser, valued at about £10, the first thing of that nature I did ever give her. Great fears we have that the plague will be a great Bill this weeke.

15th. Up by 4 o'clock and walked to Greenwich, where called at Captain Cocke's and to his chamber, he being in bed, where something put my last night's dream into my head, which I think is the best that ever was dreamt, which was that I had my Lady Castlemayne in my armes and was admitted to use all the dalliance I desired with her, and then dreamt that this could not be awake, but that it was only a dream; but that since it was a dream, and that I took so much real pleasure in it, what a happy thing it would be if when we are in our graves (as Shakespeere resembles it) we could dream, and dream but such dreams as this, that then we should not need to be so fearful of death, as we are this plague time. It was dark before I could get home, and so land at Church-yard stairs, where, to my great trouble, I met a dead corps of the plague, in the narrow ally just bringing down a little pair of stairs. But I thank God I was not much disturbed at it. However, I shall beware of being late abroad again. . . .

28th. Up, and being ready I out to Mr. Colvill, the goldsmith's, having not for some days been in the streets; but now how few people I see, and those looking like people that had taken leave of the world.

30th. Up betimes and to my business of settling my house

and papers, and then abroad and met with Hadley, our clerke, who, upon my asking how the plague goes, he told me it encreases much, and much in our parish; for, says he, there died nine this week, though I have returned [reported] but six: which is a very ill practice, and makes me think it is so in other places; and therefore the plague much greater than people take it to be. Thence, walked towards Moore-fields to see (God forbid my presumption!) whether I could see any dead corps going to the grave; but, as God would have it, did not. But, Lord! how every body's looks, and dis-course in the street is of death, and nothing else, and few people going up and down, that the towne is like a place dis-tressed and forsaken.

31st. Up; and, after putting several things in order to my removal, to Woolwich; the plague having a great encrease this week, beyond all expectation of almost 2,000, making the general Bill 7,000, odd 100; and the plague above 6,000. Thus this month ends with great sadness upon the publick, through the greatness of the plague every where through the kingdom almost. Every day sadder and sadder news of its encrease. In the City died this week 7,496, and of them 6,102 of the plague. But it is feared that the true number of the dead this week is near 10,000; partly from the poor that cannot be taken notice of, through the greatness of the num-ber, and partly from the Quakers and others that will not have any bell ring for them. Our fleete gone out to find the Dutch, we having about 100 sail in our fleete, and in them the Soveraigne one; so that it is a better fleete than the for-mer with the Duke was.

September 3rd (Lord's day). Up; and put on my coloured silk suit very fine, and my new periwigg, bought a good while since, but durst not wear, because the plague was in West-minster when I bought it; and it is a wonder what will be the fashion after the plague is done, as to periwiggs, for nobody will dare to buy any haire, for fear of the infection, that it had been cut off of the heads of people dead of the plague.

6th. Busy all the morning writing letters to several, so to dinner, to London, to pack up more things thence; and there

I looked into the street and saw fires burning in the street, as it is through the whole City, by the Lord Mayor's order.

15th. Up, it being a cold misling [misty] morning. I by water to Deptford, thinking to have seen my valentine, but I could not, and so come back again, and to the office, where a little business, and thence with Captain Cocke, and there drank a cup of good drink, which I am fain to allow myself during this plague time, by advice of all, and not contrary to my oathe, my physician being dead, an chyrurgeon [surgeon] out of the way, whose advice I am obliged to take.

19th. But, Lord! what a sad time it is to see no boats upon the River; and grass grows all up and down White Hall court, and nobody but poor wretches in the streets!

Oct. 5th. The Bill, blessed be God! is less this week by 740 of what it was the last week. Being come to my lodging I got something to eat, having eat little all the day, and so to bed, having this night renewed my promises of observing my vowes as I used to do; for I find that, since I left them off, my mind is run a' wool-gathering and my business neglected.

7th. Did business, though not much, at the office; because of the horrible crowd and lamentable moan of the poor seamen that lie starving in the streets for lack of money. Which do trouble and perplex me to the heart; and more at noon when we were to go through them, for then a whole hundred of them followed us; some cursing, some swearing, and some praying to us.

15th. (Lord's day). Up, and while I staid for the barber, tried to compose a duo of counterpoint, and I think it will do very well, it being by Mr. Berckenshaw's rule.

16th. Thence I walked to the Tower; but, Lord! how empty the streets are and melancholy, so many poor sick people in the streets full of sores; and so many sad stories overheard as I walk, every body talking of this dead, and that man sick, and so many in this place, and so many in that. And they tell me that, in Westminster, there is never a physician and but one apothecary left, all being dead; but that there are great hopes of a great decreas this week: God send it!

26th. The 'Change [stock exchange] pretty full, and the

town begins to be lively again, though the streets very empty, and most shops shut. . . .

31st. I have never lived so merrily (besides that I never got so much) as I have done this plague time, by my Lord Bruncker's and Captain Cocke's good company, and the acquaintance of Mrs. Knipp, Coleman and her husband, and Mr. Laneare, and great store of dancings we have had at my cost (which I was willing to indulge myself and wife) at my lodgings. My whole family hath been well all this while, and all my friends I know of, saving my aunt Bell, who is dead, and some children of my cozen Sarah's, of the plague. But many of such as I know very well, dead; yet, to our great joy, the town fills apace, and shops begin to be open again. Pray God continue the plague's decrease! for that keeps the Court away from the place of business, and so all goes to rack as to publick matters, they at this distance not thinking of it.

Chronology

430 B.C.
A disease epidemic strikes Athens, the ancient Greek city-state that was then fighting the Peloponnesian War against Sparta and its allies. The plague greatly weakens the Athenian army and brings about the city's permanent decline.

ca. 500–600
The Byzantine Empire suffers "Justinian's Plague," and the empire's rapid expansion comes to a halt.

1331
An epidemic of plague strikes central Asia.

1340s
The plague spreads westward along caravan routes linking central Asia with the Black Sea. At this time, the lands north of the Black Sea are controlled by the Tatars, who begin dying of plague in large numbers.

1345
The Tatars begin a siege of Kaffa, a port city on the Black Sea controlled by the Italian republic of Genoa.

1347
The plague reaches Constantinople, the capital of the Byzantine Empire. In October, Genoese merchant ships bring the plague from Kaffa to Messina, a port in Sicily, where the plague begins spreading to Italy and southern Europe.

1348
Early in the year, the plague reaches Genoa, Venice, and Florence. The epidemic quickly spreads to France, Ger-

many, Spain, and the Low Countries. The plague reaches Great Britain in the fall.

1349
The plague reaches Scotland and Ireland, as well as eastern Europe, where it begins to lose force.

1351
Under a ban of the church, the sect of flagellants, whose members did a bloody public penance in an attempt to end the plague, dies out.

1352
The plague reaches Moscow.

1361
A fresh outbreak of the bubonic plague occurs in Europe. The plague will reappear periodically throughout Europe for another four centuries. Heavy outbreaks of plague occur in Moscow in 1467, Venice in 1478, Milan and Berlin in 1576, Rome in 1591, and Venice again in 1630.

1665
The plague strikes London, prompting the king, the nobility, and many from the upper classes to flee to the countryside. The disease lasts through the summer and fall and does not abate until early 1666.

For Further Research

Books

William Bowsky, *The Black Death: A Turning Point in History?* Huntington, NY: R.E. Krieger, 1978.

Anna Montgomery Campbell, *The Black Death and Men of Learning.* New York: Columbia University Press, 1931.

Norman F. Cantor, *In the Wake of the Plague: The Black Death and the World It Made.* New York: Free Press, 2001.

Ann Carmichael, *Plague and the Poor in Renaissance Florence.* Cambridge: Cambridge University Press, 1986.

Marilyn Chase, *The Barbary Plague: The Black Death in Victorian San Francisco.* New York: Random House, 2003.

George Deaux, *The Black Death, 1347.* London: Hamilton, 1969.

Michael W. Dols, *The Black Death in the Middle East.* Princeton, NJ: Princeton University Press, 1977.

Francis Aidan Gasquet, *The Black Death of 1348 and 1349.* New York: AMS, 1977.

Robert S. Gottfried, *The Black Death: Natural and Human Disaster in Medieval Europe.* New York: Free Press, 1983.

David Herlihy, *The Black Death and the Transformation of the West.* Cambridge, MA: Harvard University Press, 1997.

Arno Karlen, *Man and Microbes: Disease and Plagues in History and Modern Times.* New York: Touchstone Books, 1996.

William McNeill, *Plagues and Peoples.* New York: Anchor Books, 1998.

Johannes Nohl, *The Black Death: A Chronicle of the Plague.* New York: J & J Harper, 1969.

Stephen Porter, *The Great Plague*. Stroud, UK: Sutton, 2000.

Barbara Tuchman, *A Distant Mirror: The Calamitous Fourteenth Century*. New York: Knopf, 1978.

Christopher Wills, *Yellow Fever, Black Goddess: The Coevolution of People and Plagues*. Cambridge, MA: Perseus, 1997.

Philip Ziegler, *The Black Death*. New York: John Day, 1969.

Websites

The Black Death, 1347–1350, www.insecta-inspecta.com. Part of a website known as "Insecta Inspecta," this page offers a complete scientific description of the rat flea that transmits the bubonic plague. The site also gives an overview of the plague's symptoms, and the effect of the Black Death on Europe's society and economy. It includes a short section of quotes from contemporary witnesses to the plague.

The Great Famine and the Black Death, www.ukans.edu/kansas/medieval/108/lectures/black_death.html. An interesting lecture by Lynn Harry Nelson of the University of Kansas on the Black Death and the famine of the early fourteenth century is posted on this page. The lecture includes maps and links to related sites, such as *The Decameron* of Boccaccio.

The Internet Medieval Sourcebook, www.fordham.edu/halsall/sbook.html. An Internet encyclopedia of original source material from the Middle Ages, with a separate section on the time of the Black Death. The Medieval Sourcebook is constantly updated with new material and includes hundreds of entries that remain impossible to find elsewhere, either in electronic or hard copy form.

Yersinia Pestis, http://members.aol.com/omaryak/plague/index.html. This short but informative page offers information on the plague bacillus, *Yersinia pestis*, and on the Black Death epidemic.

Index